Dowsing for Cures

FINDING NATURAL TREATMENTS FOR ILLNESSES

An A–Z Directory

By

Wilma Davidson

GREEN
MAGIC

Green Magic
Long Barn
Sutton Mallet
Somerset TA7 9AR
England
www.greenmagicpublishing.com

Edited by Chris Hansen

Cover Design by Rose Gotto

Typeset by Academic and Technical, Bristol
www.acadtech.co.uk

ISBN 978-0-9552908-5-5

GREEN MAGIC

CONTENTS

Dowsing for Cures has been written to give the reader information and guidelines on the art of dowsing. It is not intended as an alternative to medical advice. The author is not a qualified doctor so readers should seek advice from a medical doctor for any health problems.

I would like to say a big thank you to my children Janice, Gail and Mike who are always there offering support and to Pete Gotto and his team at Green Magic Publishing who have waved their magic wand to make the birth of this book a smooth and wonderful experience.

Wilma Davidson

INTRODUCTION

When it comes to maintaining good health, those of us who dowse have the advantage over those who have not yet learned the benefits of dowsing for health. Doctors say 'You are what you eat' and this is very true, but with the aid of a pendulum you can ensure that the food you eat is free from harmful bacteria, toxins and chemicals, and that it contains the necessary minerals and vitamins. Many illnesses are caused by a deficiency of certain minerals so your pendulum will help you to check if there is a shortage of trace minerals and can also be used to balance your energy.

To be completely healthy, the human body must be balanced in physical, emotional and spiritual energy. Listen to your body, follow your 'gut feeling' and ask your pendulum to confirm that your decision is correct. When it comes to treatment for illness, either physical or mental, go with your instincts. It's **your** body, so dowse and ask for the most beneficial treatment, whatever the health problem.

How often do you have an annoying unexplained ache or pain and wonder whether it is arthritis, bursitis or an old sports injury which has flared up? Dowsing will answer your question and enable you to diagnose the root of the problem. Dowsing can diagnose and confirm any illness and can also tell you the most beneficial treatment for the problem. Your pendulum can also confirm when plant medicine, minerals or certain metals will speed up the healing process.

The ability to dowse is rapidly becoming a necessary skill for cancer sufferers; many are exploring the alternative route, since certain cancer drugs are unavailable. BBC News today (June 14th 2007)[1] reported that certain new cancer treating drugs are so expensive that the medical profession cannot afford to purchase them. This means that patients may be forced to purchase the drugs they require to treat their cancer. One patient who was interviewed stated that he was already spending £3,000 every six weeks on the necessary drugs to fight his cancer. By dowsing, it is possible to establish which medication will fight each particular cancer and therefore avoid purchasing medication which may be of no benefit.

Ironically, our Creator has given us medicines out of the earth which centuries ago our ancestors used to treat illnesses, but sadly many of these ancient cures have been forgotten. In history we know that man has used many plants as medicines for an enormous range of illnesses and injuries. This form of treatment still exists in remote parts of the world. There are many magical plants grown in the Rainforests and although some of those are known to cure illnesses, many are not available to us. With the aid of the pendulum it is possible to channel the vibration of these precious plants to a patient with amazing results. Dowsing will confirm which plants will correctly treat the illness and also the dosage necessary. When you have mastered the art of dowsing, you will be able to diagnose illnesses **and** discover the best treatment for that particular person.

Culpepper is a fine example of a leader in this field. This famous pioneer created many remedies which are still on sale today. Perhaps it all sounds too good to be true, but this method of diagnosing illnesses and confirming treatments and cures has been used since the beginning of time. The amazing thing is that as long as you follow the basic rules, almost everyone has the ability to dowse for health.

So what are these mysterious basic rules? Simply learning to word the question correctly, cleansing the pendulum of negative energy, having permission to dowse and placing a protection around you when doing any dowsing work.

If you are concerned about a health problem, purchase an anatomy atlas which contains a page for each section of the human body. Dowse each page in turn, asking the pendulum if you are looking at the correct page for the illness. Once you have established the correct page, you will have found the section of your body that has the health problem. You are then able to dowse for the possible culprit by checking all the organs, ligaments, tendons, bones etc. in that section of the body.

When a member of your family or a friend has a heart problem, you can dowse to ask if the problem is a heart valve or a chamber. You can then use your pendulum to ask which valve or chamber is faulty and, once you have established the problem, it is time to visit your doctor. Dowsing is a gift from our Creator so enjoy it – it's there to be used.

When we fight a battle we use every piece of ammunition available to us, and the same rule applies when fighting illness and disease. Even if you don't believe that dowsing works, please dowse or ask a friend to dowse the minerals, vitamins, amino acids and plants I have suggested to find specific ones which will reduce your symptoms and bring relief.

'Your pendulum could save your life by helping you to avoid medical error' – a sweeping statement, but there is proof that a staggering number of deaths and illnesses are caused by the wrong medication or having the wrong operation. It sounds a bit far fetched, but figures show this is an everyday occurrence. Dr Mercola reports that back in 1973 when doctors in Israel staged a month long strike, the mortality rate fell by 50%. While that may not be too surprising for 1970s Israel, sadly it was not the only confirmation – a two month strike by doctors in Columbia led to a 35% reduction in deaths, and a work slow-down in Los Angeles also showed a reduction in deaths. When doctors returned to normal work schedule, death rates rose to normal figures.

You can dowse and ask your pendulum if the medical profession is responsible for a number of deaths each year, and also ask if death rate was reduced during medical doctor's strikes.

In the UK each year, roughly 1.2 million people are hospitalised due to improper medical care. Similarly, a review in the

US by Gary Null showed that 800,000 citizens died each year due to conventional medical treatment.

Perhaps the most staggering fact is that gun crime, which is a serious problem in the US, claims 40,000 lives each year. This means that three times as many deaths result from medical error.[2]

Get dowsing – with the aid of your pendulum, you may eliminate a great many health problems and avoid the possibility of medical errors!

Chart Dowsing

Some dowsers work without a chart while others prefer to hold their pendulum over a chart when dowsing. To make a medicine chart, simply draw a circle or semi-circle and divide it into a number of sections – one section for each ingredient to be dowsed.

Once you have drawn the chart and added the ingredients, whether they're plants, herbs, minerals or amino acids, start by dowsing over the chart and asking if any of the ingredients in this chart will be beneficial for the patient's illness? Ask if any of these ingredients will reduce the symptoms? If you receive a 'No' answer, it is time to check that both your pendulum and your body have been cleansed of negative energy – this negativity can influence the answers.

When the pendulum has been cleansed, hold the pendulum over each section and ask the following questions.

1. Will the supplement be beneficial to the patient's health?
2. Will it reduce symptoms?
3. Will it speed up the healing process?

Vary the questions depending on the symptoms of the illness. Everybody's body is slightly different so you will receive a 'No' answer for a few questions.

BASIC DOWSING

When you first hear about dowsing it sounds too good to be true – suddenly you are hearing details of this amazingly simple tool which can answer questions on your health problems. Perhaps the most amazing thing is that it's *free*. Even better news is that it is always available and accessible 24 hours a day, wherever you happen to be at the time.

Each time you dowse, you are using a tool that allows you to acquire information unknown to your conscious mind. The pendulum enables you access beyond your five senses – Dowsing is the only way for most of us to access the Collective Consciousness. This Collective Consciousness provides a source that can give us answers to our questions, provided they are not for self gain (i.e. the winning numbers for the lottery, or the horse who is going to win the Grand National).

Dowsing is much like any other skill – it improves with use. The more you use your pendulum or rods, the stronger the relationship you build up with your tools. When you learned to drive a car or ride a bicycle, perhaps you can remember how strange it felt. However, quickly the act becomes automatic and almost an extension of yourself – you no longer have to think about when to change gear, etc. The same thing happens with dowsing. Once you start dowsing regularly and learn to trust your pendulum, you will build up a relationship and will know when the correct answer is given. You will thank your pendulum for saving you money. It will guide you to purchase the correct medication and so avoid buying pills and potions which will not be beneficial.

Learning to dowse involves using the right side of the brain to communicate with the universal knowledge we all possess. In normal, everyday life we cannot access this great pool of

1

information and most of us never learn how to, unless we become very experienced in meditation. Your pendulum will enable you to bridge the invisible gap between you and the infinite intelligence. Even those of us who were always at the bottom of the class at school and absolutely useless at passing exams on basic or academic subjects will be able to dowse to access this gigantic pool of knowledge.

The only skills needed to dowse are the ability to clear your mind of other subjects when asking a question, and being both mentally and emotionally stable. It's not good to dowse when you feel depressed, as you can pass your negative energy to the pendulum which will affect the accuracy of the answers. Please don't doubt your dowsing ability. Most people can master the art of dowsing given a little time. I have taught this subject at Adult classes and found all pupils could quickly master this art.

Dowsing is a wonderful tool to enable us to heal our body. Within each living being, whether human or animal, there is a basic knowledge of everything which is taking place in our body. This knowledge includes an ongoing analysis of the mineral balance in the body, where there is a deficiency, and what to eat to correct the imbalance.

How often have you had an unexplained urge to eat a certain food? Cravings are your body guiding you to a source of minerals where there is a shortage. When you have a notion to eat a banana then your body is probably deficient in potassium. If you have a desire for spinach, your body may be low in iron.

Animals are a fine example of this. They seem naturally able to tap into this store of knowledge and know when to eat certain plants or grass to give their body extra minerals or vitamins.

Dowsers are often asked if the church disapproves of dowsing and if using the pendulum is evil. Well, the church does not disapprove of dowsing and proof of this is found many years ago – Abbe Mermet was given the Pope's blessing and invited to visit the Vatican in order to assist in the planning and restoration of the Cathedral of St. Peter. That's certainly good proof that the Catholic Church accepts dowsing when used for good.[3]

Rolf Gordon, in his book 'Are you Sleeping in a Safe Place' reports that The Roman Catholic church decreed back in 1942 that if a Christian wants to do God's work and help himself and others by dowsing, this work is blessed by the Church, but it should not be used solely for gain.[6]

Further proof comes from the Holy Bible. Dowsing Rods are mentioned in many pages and in Exodus 4.17 'Oppression of the Israelites,' God tells Moses 'And Thou Shalt Take This Rod in Thine Hand Wherewith thou Shalt do Signs.' This excerpt provides proof not only that God approved of Dowsing, but also that Moses was a Dowser![4]

Dowsers are often asked the question 'Does it really work? Is it magic? Is it a spirit somewhere in space giving the answers, or is it quantum physics?' No one really knows the correct answer, but we do know that it works. German researchers drilling in Sri Lanka found that, over 691 drillings, dowsers were 96% correct, whereas only an estimated 30 to 50% were correct when using conventional methods.[5]

The Pendulum

You can dowse using either a pendulum or dowsing rods, but if you are a beginner I recommend using a pendulum. It's very simple to use and fits comfortable into your pocket. Your pendulum can be any small weighted object, preferably round or oval so that its weight is balanced on both sides. There is no need to purchase an expensive crystal pendulum as you can dowse just as effectively with a Yale key attached to a piece of string. Perhaps you may prefer to make your own pendulum from a stone found on the beach or a favourite pendant – whatever you use it will work, provided the base is heavier than the chain. When out on walks with my dog, I have often used the dog's lead to get an answer to a question. You can use any tool, so long as it is heavy enough to swing!

Enthusiastic dowsers often make their own pendulum and rods. When purchasing a pendulum, you will find that you are drawn to one particular stone – that is the right one for you. You'll probably become aware that, although several stones look almost exactly identical, there is one stone that feels much more friendly and comfortable than the others. Don't dither! Purchase this pendulum.

I am often asked if it's important which hand we use to hold the pendulum. The answer is no! If you are more comfortable holding the pendulum in your right hand, or left hand, then that is the best hand for you to use for dowsing. It doesn't matter which hand you use. The energy will come through when you use your intent to dowse.

Learning the Dowsing Language

Dowsing is a two way communication between you and your pendulum, so you need to know the language. Fortunately there are only three important signs to learn and once you have mastered these signs, all that's needed is some practice.

When you ask the pendulum a question, you will receive a 'Yes,' 'No' or 'Don't Know' sign. Here are the simple rules to find your pendulum's signs and allow you to communicate with it.

Sit down and relax. Mentally send a bright white light through the pendulum to cleanse it of negative energy. This is important, as pendulums purchased from a store may have been handled by many folks and some could have acquired negative energy.

Hold the pendulum with a chain of any length between 3 to 8 inches. A longer chain is more difficult to control. Start by swinging the pendulum very slightly to get it moving then ask it to please show you your 'Yes' sign. This may be a clockwise circle, an anti-clockwise circle or back and forward. Please don't think it is not working if your sign is different from your friend's sign, as we all have our own signs.

Once you have a positive 'Yes' sign it is time to learn your 'No' sign. Ask your pendulum to please show you your 'No' sign. Again, this can be any one of the above listed signs. When the pendulum has given you your 'No' sign it is time to establish your 'Don't' Know' sign.

The 'Don't Know' sign is very important as it is the sign used when you have phrased a question wrongly, or asked a question which you are not entitled to know the answer. i.e., 'Is my neighbour having an affair with the milkman?'

The 'Don't Know' sign may also be used when you ask a question which will affect your freewill. We are all born with freewill so the pendulum will often refuse to answer this type of question. If you ask 'Should I take extra iron?' it will not answer – you have the freewill to choose whether you take it or not. You must phrase the question differently. You should ask 'Is my body short of iron?' or 'Will my body benefit from a supplement of iron?'

To find your 'Don't Know' sign, start by mentally asking the pendulum to show you this sign and watch with interest to see what happens. Some folks report their pendulum goes on strike and firmly refuses to answer a question which is wrongly worded, so if this happens please don't think your pendulum is not working! Your 'Don't Know' sign may be a swing at 45% or straight back and forward. Ask several times to be shown each sign so that the answers are consistent. For the first few weeks when you start dowsing it is wise to ask the pendulum to show you your signs, but after a short period this is no longer necessary unless you're using a different pendulum.

When you have established your signs there are some basic rules to remember when you dowse.

1. Always place a light of protection around you before you start to dowse, as this protects you from the presence of any negative energy.
2. Always mentally run a beam of white light of healing energy through your pendulum to cleanse it of negative energy before asking questions, and again when you have finished using it.
3. The late Terry Ross devised three questions which serious dowsers ask before dowsing a question.

(a) CAN I? This is asking whether or not you are a good channel to dowse. Perhaps you are tired or ill?
(b) MAY I? is asking permission to dowse. Perhaps it is not right to dowse this question about a person.
(c) SHOULD I? Is it a suitable time? The energy could be wrong or another factor could influence results.

Once you become an experienced dowser, you may find that you unconsciously tune in to your pendulum and know the answer before the pendulum starts to move. Some dowsers report a tingling in one finger or an ear. I get a tingling almost like needles and pins running up one side of my right hand, from the tip of my smallest finger, when the answer is 'Yes'. Sometimes I am convinced I can feel excitement coming from the pendulum, as though it is pleased I asked that particular question.

Please remember it is important not to dowse if you are feeling very tired, depressed, worried, afraid or sad, as your negative energy will be passed to the pendulum and you will get wrong answers. For this reason I repeat it is very important to cleanse the pendulum each time you use it.

Warning – Don't influence the pendulum. It is very easy to be so over enthusiastic about the answer to a question that you are mentally saying to the pendulum 'please, please don't say No'. It's important to check your thoughts when the answer is very important to you.

A good reminder is to say the words used by many dowsers 'Let this by *Thy* Will and not *My* Will.'

Phrasing the question correctly

Please think carefully about the wording of a question before you dowse. It is often a good idea to phrase the question in several different ways. If you get the same answer, then you know it is correct.

I had an example of how easy it is to make a mistake when asking a question of the pendulum this week. A friend's daughter had collapsed unconscious on the floor and been taken into the local hospital.

I was told by my spirit doctors that she was sleeping over Geopathic Stress. This is caused by negative energy from underground rivers, which weakens the immune system. I dowsed and asked my pendulum if the girl was sleeping over Geopathic Stress energy and received a firm No from the pendulum. This answer confused me as I was convinced that this negative energy had been the root cause of her illness, but each time I asked the question I received a firm NO. The question still niggled in my mind when I was in bed and suddenly I realised I had asked the wrong question – I had asked if she is sleeping over this harmful energy, when she is of course now sleeping in a hospital bed where this negative energy is not present. When I rephrased the question and asked if there was Geopathic Stress present in her home, I received a Yes answer. I then asked if the girl had been sleeping over a Geopathic Stress line and received a positive Yes answer, which reminded me that it is easy to rush and ask a question without stopping to think if the wording is correct.

Dowsing for health problems

You can use your pendulum to diagnose an area in the body where a health problem is situated. A simple exercise is to ask the person to lie on a bed or the floor and hold the pendulum over their body.

Mentally ask the pendulum to show you the 'Yes' sign when the pendulum passes over a trouble area. Start by holding the pendulum over the patient's head and then slowly move it down the length of the body to the feet. The pendulum will swing and give you the 'Yes' sign when it passes over an organ which is not functioning properly, or an area where an energy blockage or imbalance is present.

Another method of locating a health problem area is to write a list of the body's main organs and glands and move the pendulum over each item on the list while asking by name if each one is balanced.

Once you have made a list and dowsed to locate problem areas, you can then check each problem area on a 1 to 10 scale. As pain can often be deflected from another area, it is important to find the source of the problem – for example, shoulder and neck pain can both be caused by wear at the top of the spine. It's important to diagnose the source of the problem before trying to find the right medication for the trouble.

To check on a 1–10 scale you write a list of the numbers with number 1 at the bottom of the scale and number 10 at the top of the scale. You then ask if the problem is above five on the scale of seriousness, and if you receive a No answer you can ask if it is above 3 on the scale.

If you get a 'No' answer then you know that this is a minor health issue. The pendulum will show you all areas of the body where there are problems, so some may be very minor. However, as we have asked it to show us all health problems, it will do its job and show us each problem.

You can be more specific in your question by asking to be shown any established health problem areas, or any areas which require treatment.

Take time experimenting. Ask several questions and you will, by a process of elimination, receive accurate information about major and minor illnesses.

Once you have located the health problems, it's time to dowse to find any mineral and vitamin deficiencies and perhaps discover which plant medicine may be beneficial to expedite healing and reduce symptoms. When you have used your pendulum to dowse if the medication will be beneficial to the health complaint, you then need to dowse to find the correct amount to take (i.e., one teaspoonful, one drop etc.). The next step is to establish how often this medication should be taken each day. Ask your pendulum whether the medication is required – (1) once each day, (2) twice each day, (3) three times each day. When you have received the correct answer it is time to check whether this medication should be taken (1) before food, (2) with food, (3) after food.

Some of these medications may only be required for a few days in order to regain the correct level in the body, so dowse and ask if the medication is required for (1) more than three days, (2) more than seven days, (3) more than ten days. These dowsing questions apply to plant medicine, amino acids, vitamins, minerals or metals. You can also use your pendulum to transform any negative energy to positive energy in a matter of minutes.

Dowsers often say that they are very much like doctors, with a different and much simpler medicine kit. This is very true; the dowser has the advantage over the doctor in that he does not need to know the person's symptoms to be able to diagnose the illness. By mentally asking a few questions, he can locate the illness and find the best treatment.

Please don't worry if you are unable to dowse, as dowsing is taught at some adult centres and there are dowsing groups in many parts of the world that will be able to help you. Details of Dowsing Societies are listed in the Reference section and the British Society of Dowsers will be pleased to give you contact details of your nearest group where you can learn this skill. If you prefer to delegate, you can use the services of a radiesthesia therapist.

Radiesthesia

Radiesthesia is the name given to medical dowsing and, as Shakespeare said so long ago 'There is more to heaven than ever you dream.' It's very true in this case, as most folks admit it has never entered their mind to consider the possibility of using radiesthesia to heal the sick.

So what exactly is this method of treatment? Radiesthesia is often practised by therapists who have knowledge of the body and are experienced dowsers. Some use a specimen to dowse over in order to help them to diagnose an illness, perhaps a piece of the patient's hair or a nail clipping as a witness. Others place a sample in a small envelope called a 'Witness' envelope and dowse over the envelope. Whatever method is used, the result should be the same.

My first experience of this form of dowsing was thirty years ago when I visited a homeopathic doctor for a shoulder injury. To my astonishment the first question this doctor asked was 'Do you Dowse?' I looked at her in astonishment and asked why she needed to know this information. She explained that my body needed slightly different medicine every day, so she would dowse to find three medicines suitable for treating my shoulder and· I was to dowse each morning in order to ascertain which medication was needed that day.

When I got home and digested this information, I realised that it made a lot of sense. The body's energy is different each day, depending on the food we've eaten and other factors.

So 'What is Radiesthesia and how does it work?' The answer you receive depends on which dowser you ask! Is it a phenomenon which can only be explained by the laws of physics, or is it man's ability to link into the Universal Medical Register? You can dowse and ask if, with the aid of the pendulum, dowsers are able to create a direct link with the Universal Medical Register? You can then ask if the pendulum can be used to channel healing energy to a patient?

We are all made of energy, so is radiesthesia simply a way of using our energy to link into another vibration? Perhaps your pendulum will confirm the answer.

References

1. BBC Television News 14th June 2007.
2. Dr Jospeh Mercola, 'When Doctors Strike, Fewer People Die' June 3rd www.mercola.com
3. Kathe Bachler *Earth Radiation* published by Wordmaster 1989. page 51 Source Abbe Mermet *The Dowser, Himself a Scientific Instrument.* Alsatia publisher.
4. The Holy Bible. Old & New Testament. 1958. Collins Clear Type Press.
5. Primrose Cooper, *The Healing Power of Light.* Piatkus. ISBN 0 7499 2069 6.
6. Rolf Gordon. *Are You Sleeping in a Safe place.* Available from Dulwich Health, 130 Gipsy Hill, London SE19 1PL.

ABSCESS

Anyone who has suffered an abscess will tell you it's a pain on the butt! And why does it so often occur on the buttocks? An abscess is a painful localised ball of puss which can appear in any of a number of areas in the body. Today, many folks get antibiotics to clear the poison, but there are some good old fashioned cures which are perhaps better for long term health.

When a cabbage leaf with its central stem removed is placed on a wound overnight, it will act like a poultice and draw the poison out of the body. When I was a youngster my mother used to place a wet piece of bread with baking soda on the infected area and leave it there for several hours in order to draw out the poison.

Dowse and ask if your body is short of Zinc, as this mineral is a great healer. Also, Dowse and ask your pendulum if Beta carotene taken 4 times a day will be beneficial, as it's recommended by some folks.

Bathing the wound with Colloidal silver will kill any harmful bacteria and enable the abscess to heal more quickly. Dowse and ask if your body would benefit from a supplement of Sulphur, as this mineral cleanses the blood. Also dowse to ask the pendulum if you are sleeping over Geopathic Stress, as this can lower the immune system. Abscesses usually only occur when your immune system is low, so dowse and ask if your body would benefit from a course of multi minerals and vitamins? If you regularly suffer from abscesses, it is wise to dowse to find the cause of these painful outbreaks. Your pendulum will confirm the best treatment for this painful point and will confirm the cause.

ACID/ALKALINE LEVEL IN YOUR BODY

The acid/alkaline level of your body's fluids has a big impact on your health, so it's important to keep an eye on this level to avoid all sorts of health problems which seem linked to an imbalance.

What is the pH balance of your body? And what is pH? It stands for Potential of Hydrogen and is the way we measure the body's Acid/Alkaline level. The lower the pH on the scale, the more acid there is. The usual way to measure the pH level is on a 1–14 scale, so below 7 is acidic and above is alkaline. Some charts work on a 1–10 scale but however you measure the level, the acid content should be lower than the alkaline level.

When the pH is unbalanced, more often than not it is too acidic rather than too alkaline. Acidosis is linked to certain illnesses, including bladder and kidney problems, cardio-vascular problems and osteoporosis. If your acid level is too high, you may well suffer from digestive problems, low energy level or weight problems. Digestive problems and stomach disorders are often caused by an imbalance of acids and alkaline pH in your body so dowse and ask:

1. Are your digestive problems caused by an acid/alkaline imbalance?
2. Does your body have an excess Acid level?
3. Will more alkaline food in your diet improve the symptoms?

The easiest way to keep the pH balance level is to make a conscious effort to eat more fruit and vegetables to counteract the effect of proteins and sugars. Acid forming foods include fish, seafood, poultry, meat, eggs, dairy food, grains, alcohol, sweets and cakes while alkaline forming foods include most fruits, vegetables, seeds and spices.

You will be amazed how much better you feel when you increase the level of fruit and vegetables in your diet. You will probably notice the improvement very quickly.

Skin brushing

Skin brushing may sound a little strange, but the skin is the body's largest organ and sheds pounds of acid each day through its pores. By brushing the skin each morning you effectively remove acid and dead skin and allow the skin to eliminate more acid.

You should use a long handled natural bristle brush and it doesn't matter which direction you brush in, as long as you do some skin brushing. After a short period you will start to feel benefit. You can brush all areas of your choice but avoid brushing your face as the skin is delicate. Dowse and ask the following questions:

1. Would your health benefit from brushing your skin each day?
2. Will skin brushing remove some acid from your skin?
3. Is brushing your skin for two minutes each day sufficient to remove acidic toxins from the skin?

The first time you brush your skin it feels a bit foreign, but after a few days you begin to enjoy it and feel benefit, so try it. You'll be glad you've become a skin brusher!

ACNE

Acne is a common complaint in puberty. As it occurs at an age when we lack self confidence, having a large number of inflamed spots on your face is a real embarrassment. It's caused by a disorder of the sebaceous glands and when these glands become inflamed, skin eruption follows.

Dowse and ask if any of the following Homeopathic remedies would improve the acne – (1) Belladonna, (2) Pulsatilla, (3) Silicea, (4) Sulphur, (5) Hepar Sulph, or (6) Kali Bromatum.

Ask if bathing the face in Colloidal Silver will reduce infection? This natural antibiotic will kill harmful bacteria on your skin. Tea Tree is one of Mother Nature's natural antibiotics, so dowse and ask if bathing with Tee Tree oil will destroy micro-organisms and reduce symptoms. Propolis is a natural healer, so dowse and ask if this anti-inflammatory cream would reduce the Acne on your skin. Ask your pendulum if a multi mineral supplement which includes Sulphur would be beneficial?

There are many natural products which can help to reduce the symptoms of Acne, so dowse and find out which ones will best benefit you.

ADD AND ADHD

Scientists used to believe that while a baby was in its mother's womb, it was protected from environmental toxins and chemicals. Alas, they are now very aware that this is not the case.

The Environmental Working Group commissioned tests on ten cord Blood samples and as you can imagine, they all contained a lot of nasty stuff!

Each cord tested contained an average of 200 contaminants in their blood – what a start to life! These contaminants included mercury, fire retardants, pesticides and the Teflon chemical PFDA.

The blood samples tested were from babies born in hospital and scientists tested for 413 industrial and consumer product chemicals.[59] Is it any wonder there is an increase in the number of children suffering from ADHD, Autism and other health problems, when their blood has been bombarded with pollution since they were conceived? A high percentage of the chemicals in all the cosmetics you use soak through your skin into your blood. When you are pregnant these chemicals travel on to the placenta and to the baby in the womb. Dowse and ask the following questions:

1. Did my baby receive any chemicals from my blood when in the womb?
2. Did these chemicals affect his or her health?

Reliable Proof that some symptoms of ADHD can be linked to chemicals and heavy metals in the diet comes from The Hyperactive Children's Support Group, who report that 89% of children diagnosed with ADHD showed a reduction in symptoms when artificial colours were removed from their diet.[57] Well done to 'Smarties,' who've taken the troublesome colours from their sweets. And they still taste good!

The Food Commission in UK reported that most additives are banned from food and drinks eaten by young children and babies, yet many medicines for this age group contain an alarming cocktail of these same additives which are banned from their food. It doesn't make any sense that children are being fed medication which contains banned chemicals.

What happens when these chemicals interact with chemicals passed from the mother when in the womb? It's a minefield. Dowse and ask the following:

1. Are any of your child's symptoms linked to chemicals in their blood?
2. Are any of the child's symptoms linked to heavy metals in their blood?

The Food Magazine surveyed 41 medicines sold for consumption by the under 3 years age group, and what did the survey expose? Four Azo dye colourings, eight Benzoate, two Sulphite preservatives and six Sweeteners, all of which are banned from food and drink for the under 3 year olds. The alarming fact is that those products surveyed were cough mixtures, teething gels and junior Paracetemol etc., many of which are given to a child when their immune system is low.

Colouring Additives are banned from food and drink for children under 3 years, but an abundance was found in the tested products and only one item gave a warning that E124 may cause allergic reactions including Asthma.

Artificial Sweeteners are also banned from food and drink in this age group as sweeteners Sorbitol, Maltitol and Xylitol can have a laxative effect and this symptom is certainly not welcome, particularly when the child is feeling low.

Preservatives are another group which were also banned. However, a range of these banned preservatives were found in the medicines. Some gave a warning that the preservative could have unpleasant side effects, e.g. may irritate the eyes, skin and mucus surfaces. One preservative carried a warning that a symptom could be contact Dermatitis.[57] Dowse and ask the following questions:

1. Does the teething gel contain any banned chemicals?

2. Does the Junior Paracetemol contain any banned chemicals?
3. Does the cough mixture contain any banned chemicals?
4. Do any of these products contain chemicals which will affect the child's behaviour?

Does your child have sufficient essential fatty acids in their diet? The Physiology & Behavior Magazine reported the results of research on the levels of essential fatty acids in boys 6–12 years. Those boys with lower levels of Omega 3 fatty acid concentration suffered more health problems, including temper tantrums, sleep problems, antibiotic use and colds.[66] Dowse and ask the following questions:

1. Does my child have sufficient level of essential fatty acids in his diet?
2. Would a supplement of Omega 3 in his diet reduce some of the ADHD symptoms?
3. Would a supplement of Omega 3 improve his health?

Omega 3 benefits the health of most folks, so dowse and ask if your own body is short of this essential fatty acid. Also, dowse and ask if the child would benefit from a low phosphorous diet?

Many mothers report that their child's behaviour deteriorates when they have eaten certain foods and are convinced that certain foods trigger ADHD symptoms, so dowse and ask if the following foods or mineral deficiencies have an adverse effect on the child.

1. Can cheese aggravate the symptoms?
2. Does Cows Milk, which has several times more phosphorous than human milk, aggravate their symptoms?
3. Do Cola and other fizzy drinks affect behaviour?
4. Does the child have a Magnesium deficiency?
5. Are levels of Copper too high in the child's body?
6. Does the child suffer mood swings? If so, dowse and ask if Seratonin or Tryptophan will reduce the mood swings.
7. Does the child have a deficiency of Iron?
8. Is the child's body low in Iodine? If you receive a 'Yes' answer, dowse and ask if the Thyroid gland is dysfunctional.

All children need slightly different treatments as their bodies are short of different minerals, so dowse and ask which of the above items may be beneficial to your child.

AGEING

Many of us worry about getting old and the signs of ageing, but it is possible to keep age at bay by having a good healthy diet and taking certain minerals and plants. Wild Yam is the favourite. Dowse and ask if this plant will slow the ageing process in your body? Make sure you cleanse your pendulum before you ask the question, as the wrong answer could be devastating!

AIDS

AIDs is a bit of a mystery illness. There are so many conflicting theories about the cause and treatment of this dreadful illness. As it is linked to a weak immune system, it's important to take note of the several natural products that help to build up this important system.

Dowse and ask if the patient's body is short of Selenium. The AIDs virus is known to cause a shortage of this mineral.

AIDs sufferers are usually deficient in several minerals and respond well to plant medication, so dowse the following list and ask which ones will be beneficial. Start by asking if any of the items on the list would be beneficial to the patient's health? When you receive a 'Yes' sign, ask a separate question for each one on the list, and you may find that you receive confirmation to more than one item. (1) Lapacho, (2) Echinacea, (3) Glutathione, (4) Clover, (5) Feverfew, (6) Thyme, (7) Melatonin, or (8) Myrrh.

Zinc increases T-cell function. A deficiency of Zinc causes loss of T-cells in animals, so dowse and ask the following questions.

1. Is there a Zinc deficiency in the AIDs sufferer?
2. Is their body deficient in Vitamin B6?
3. Is their body deficient of iron?

4. Would they benefit from a supplement of the amino acids Cysteine or Tryptophan?
5. Dowse and ask if their Pineal Gland is out of balance and if it would benefit from Healing.

Many of the above have been found beneficial to certain sufferers, so get dowsing. The most effective way to deal with this illness is to keep the immune system very strong.

ALLERGIES

An allergic reaction is an abnormal sensitivity which occurs when your body's immune system reacts to certain substances. Often it is a reaction to the most unlikely one, and the source of these adverse reactions can be a mystery.

The reaction can be caused by a range of substances including certain foods, colorants, animal fur, perfume or something in the environment. Whatever the root of the allergy, your pendulum will be able to locate the culprit. If you find it impossible to dowse or do not have confidence in your dowsing ability, don't despair. Many chemists offer an approved test.

What is an allergen? It is any substance which can instigate an unhealthy allergic reaction in your body. Almost everybody is allergic to something, but many of us are fortunate enough to go through life without ever experiencing an allergic reaction, while others have Big Problems.

There are many simple explanations for some of the causes of allergic reaction. One culprit can be a high level of histamine in your body, so dowse and ask if your body has a high level of histamine.

Another reason can be an imbalance in the Acid/Alkaline level in your body, as this will create digestive problems when you eat certain foods. Don't persevere if you get an adverse reaction to certain foods, no matter how much you love them – always listen to your body. The symptoms are warning you that this food is a 'No Go Area'.

If you have in the past suffered from a severe viral infection, it is quite possible that it has caused damage to your body's immune system. A weakness in your immune system will make you more sensitive to certain allergens, so this is a question for the pendulum. Perhaps your body would benefit from a short course of the plant Echinacea, which is renowned for strengthening the immune system?

Dowse the following questions:

1. Do I have an allergic reaction to dairy products?
2. Do I have an allergic reaction to organic cow's milk?
3. Is my Adrenal Gland balanced?
4. Is the Acid/Alkaline level correct?
5. Does my body have excess mercury?
6. Does my body have excess Histamine?
7. Is my spleen correctly balanced?
8. Would my spleen benefit from a boost of healing energy?

You can also dowse and ask your pendulum if any of the following supplements would benefit your body. Ask each item separately by name and phrase the questions differently. (1) Echinacea, (2) Cat's Claw, or (3) Quercetin (*a natural anti histamine*).

Is my body deficient in any of the following minerals, metals or vitamins? (1) Manganese, (2) Magnesium, (3) MSM, (4) Zinc, (5) Iron, (6) Vit B6, (7) Vit B12, or (8) Germanium (*improves oxygen*). If you receive a 'Yes' answer, dowse each separately.

An allergic reaction to soy can be the cause of many health problems, including bed wetting, sleep disturbances, sinus trouble, ear infection, joint pains, chronic fatigue, unexplained coughing, hives, a swollen tongue or anaphylactic shock. Although we don't hear much about the possibility of an allergy to soy, it is one of the 'Big Eight' allergens; peanuts and soy are members of the same botanical family.[14] Dowse and ask if your symptoms are caused by an allergic reaction to soy?

If you suffer regularly from skin irritation, runny nose or itchy eyes, perhaps your symptoms are linked to an Acid/Alkaline imbalance. These symptoms can be the body's way of dealing with an excess acid level. Dowse and ask the following questions:

1. Are my allergy symptoms linked to an acid/alkaline imbalance?
2. Does my body have excess acid level?
3. Dowse on a 1–10 scale to ask the level of acid pH in the body? Your acid level should not be higher than your alkaline level.

Food Intolerance affects literally millions of people and it can often be a slow process to find the culprit, so this is another situation in which dowsing is invaluable.

Ask your pendulum if the food which has caused the reaction was eaten less than three days ago? (*Please remember to cleanse your pendulum before starting the exercise to ensure the correct answers.*) If the answer is 'Yes' you can then ask if it was eaten within the last twenty four hours? If you get a 'Yes' answer once more, you can ask if it was eaten within the past twelve hours, and when you get confirmation of roughly when this food was eaten, you can make a list of all the food and drink you consumed in that period and dowse to ask which is the culprit.

To speed up the exercise, you can ask if the allergen is one of the first five foods on your list and if you get a 'No' answer, you know not to waste energy asking about these foods and to move on to the next five foods.

Dowse and ask the pendulum if more than one of the foods on the list is an allergen? Once you have established which food or drink is the culprit, you can then check the ingredients in the food and dowse to find which ingredient is causing the reaction. You can dowse each chemical in the item and, by a process of elimination, you will quickly find the allergen.

If you are not confident about dowsing for the cause of the problem, you may prefer another method which is available through a Lloyds pharmacist. Lloyds offer a Food Intolerance Testing Service in UK, whereby you have a tiny sample of blood taken which is analysed by York test laboratories. The exercise involves the multi allergy screening test of allergic reaction to 36 of the most common food and airborne allergens.[15] Similar services will be available in other countries. Dowse and ask if this test will locate your allergen.

Could your allergy symptoms be caused by fitted carpets in your home? According to experts at the Healthy Flooring Network, fitted carpets are a prime culprit in the rise of allergies and asthma as they are home to millions of dust mites. Dowse and ask your pendulum if any of your allergy symptoms are linked to dust mites in your carpets?

Now dowse and ask if dust mites are the prime cause of your symptoms? You can have multiple allergies so it's important to ask if this is the sole cause of the symptoms. If dust mites are indeed the sole cause then, while it's a depressing thought if you have spent a lot of money on good quality carpets, at least you know the cause of the discomfort.

ALOPECIA

Alopecia causes embarrassment, as it creates patches of hair loss and can be bad for self esteem. There are a few possible causes but usually it is linked to a mineral deficiency or an underactive thyroid.

Zinc is a wonderful healer and this mineral plays an important part in creating healthy skin and hair, while also healing wounds. Perhaps you remember your mother producing the jar of Zinc and Castor oil ointment to heal cuts and scrapes when you were a child. Zinc tablets are available from health shops, but I recommend purchasing a brand which contains a small level of copper.

Many Alopecia sufferers have a Kelp deficiency. Dowse and ask the pendulum the following questions:

1. Is your body is short of Kelp?
2. Is your body short of Iodine?
3. Ask if your thyroid gland is balanced.

4. Ask the pendulum if your Alopecia would be improved by a course of hypnotherapy?
5. Are you sleeping over Geopathic Stress?

Research at the Free University in Brussels showed that certain patients suffering from this auto immune disease responded very well to a course of hypnotherapy. After three sessions, some patients experienced hair growth. It's well worth dowsing to ask if your symptoms would respond to this painless therapy.[11]

As doctors state that this is an auto immune illness, it's a good idea to build up the immune system. Dowse and ask if your body would benefit from taking a course of Echinacea, as this natural medication is well known as a friend to the immune system.

One of the biggest enemies of our immune system is Geopathic Stress, so it is important to dowse to check for the presence of this unwelcome energy.

ALZHEIMER'S DISEASE

Alzheimer's disease affects the brain of sufferers. This progressive disease is characterized by a noticeable disturbance in the brain which affects speech and memory. So, what is the root cause of this dreadful debilitating illness which disrupts the quality of life and takes away our dignity?

Some scientists believe this illness is linked to an increase in the production or accumulation of the protein Beta-Amyloid, which leads to nerve cell death. This in turn causes deficits in the neuro-transmitters, which are the brains messengers; when this department goes wrong, messages get scrambled.[19]

Excess levels of Amyloid B protein seem to trigger production of Free Radicals, which in turn seem to lead to more Amyloid B. This is thought to be a major factor in brain disorders like Alzheimer's. Research has shown that the higher the level of Amyloids, the more advanced the illness.[35]

There is not yet sufficient research results to prove conclusively that this is the correct explanation for the illness, but let's dowse and ask if an increase in the production of the protein Beta-amyloid is responsible for some Alzheimer's symptoms?

Dowse and ask if the body is short of any of the following. (Also ask if it has an excess.)

1. Does your body have the correct level of DMAE? This is the most important nutrient – brain chemical – acetye-choline.
2. Would you benefit from a supplement of Lecithen granules?
3. Does your body have excess lead?
4. Does your body have excess Aluminium?
5. Does your body have excess Mercury from Amalgam fillings?
6. Does your body have excess Manganese?
7. Dowse if the A1 Receptor working is too slow – can serotonin help?
8. Would a supplement of any of the following items benefit your health? (1) Selenium, (2) Gingko Biloba, (3) Evening Primrose, (4) Fish oil, (5) Boron, (6) Magnesium, (7) Niacin Zinc, (8) Chromium, (9) Cobalt, (10) B12, (11) Riboflavin, (12) Niacin, (13) Folic Acid, (14) Taurine, (15) Molybdenum, (16) Iodine or (17) Copper?
9. Do I have an impaired glucose transporter? If you receive a 'Yes' answer, ask the pendulum to please repair the glucose level.
10. Do you have a deficiency of Tocophgroll? (*Vitamin E*)
11. Would a supplement of Ascorbic acid help if it is channelled to the brain?

Alzheimer's disease claims many lives worldwide. In the US, 100,000 lives each year are lost to this illness. There are 4.5 million sufferers in the USA and it is the fourth highest cause of death; half of all nursing home beds are claimed by Alzheimer's patients, so there is an urgent need to find a cure for these sufferers.

New research published in Molecular Biology reveals Delta 9 – Tetrahydro cannabis, an active compound in the well known plant marijuana, can inhibit the enzyme AchE which is linked to the cause of the disease. It can unblock the formation of brain-clogging amyloid plaque in parts of the brain important for memory and cognition.[65]

Recent research in California on the effect of the curry spice Turmeric on Alzheimer's Disease showed interesting results. The chemical Bisdemethoxycurcum in Turmeric has the ability to enable macrophlanges in the patients blood to get rid of the brain plaque protein called amyloid beta. Curcumin root has been used in natural treatment for many centuries, so it's good news that researchers have found a chemical in this plant that can possibly help to reduce symptoms of Alzheimer's Disease.

If you know of anyone who suffers from Alzheimer's Disease, dowse and ask if this chemical in Turmeric can help to reduce their symptoms? If you receive a 'Yes' answer, then ask the pendulum how often they need to eat a meal containing Turmeric to reduce the symptoms. You can then dowse and ask the level required, i.e. is one half of a level teaspoonful of this spice each day sufficient to reduce symptoms? You can then ask if less is required, or ask if more is required?

It is important to ask if this spice will cause any harmful side effects, or if it will interact badly with any of medication being taken. An interesting thought is – 'If the spice Turmeric can help reduce the symptoms of Alzheimer's Disease, does this mean that folks who regularly eat curried food will have less symptoms?'[71]

There has been a lot of talk over the years about aluminium in the body being a cause of Alzheimer's and this is confirmed in autopsy reports: Dr Russell Blaylock reports that 70% of patients studied had a higher level of aluminium in their brain. Aluminium has been found in the body of patients who have died of both Alzheimer's disease and of Parkinson's disease, so how does this aluminium get into their body? That's the mystery.

There are several explanations – if the patient suffered from indigestion or heartburn for a long period of time, the source could be antacids. Many brands contain a small amount of aluminium.

Many modern deodorants also contain aluminium, so purchase a brand which is aluminium-free from your local health shop.

The finger is pointing firmly at Aluminium as a positive link with the increase in cases of both Alzheimer's disease and senile dementia. Research has repeatedly shown abnormally high levels of aluminium in those patient's brains. Could another source be aluminium cooking pots and kitchen utensils?

Many old cookware used on electric cookers contained aluminium. I found this out the hard way; when I was a young bride, I was concerned about cleaning my lovely engagement ring. Someone advised me to place it in a pot of boiling water with some washing soda. I followed their instructions and disaster struck as the washing soda took the aluminium lining off the pot and my ring ended up covered in a grey scum. When I complained to them about the result, they pointed out that they had said baking soda and not washing soda!

Dowse and ask if the presence of aluminium in the brain affects the working of the brain? Next, dowse and ask if aluminium in the brain contributes to Alzheimer's disease? Ask your pendulum if it is better for health to avoid aluminium cookware.

Norway's Central Board of Statistics states there is a direct link between aluminium in drinking water and dementia.[32] Dowse and ask if aluminium in drinking water can have a detrimental effect on the brain? Next, ask if aluminium in deodorants can soak into your blood stream? It is important to be aware of these possible health hazards which are part of everyday living.

We hear that brain diseases including Alzheimer's disease, dementia and brain tumours are on the increase, but what most of us don't realise is the gigantic scale of the increase. In the past 25 years, brain diseases have increased by 300% in countries where the artificial sweetener Aspartame is used. Is this simply a coincidence, or is there a link between this artificial sweetener and brain diseases?[31] Dowse and ask your pendulum if Aspartame in the diet is linked to any brain illnesses? Then ask if regularly eating food containing Aspartame can cause brain illnesses?

Food for thought is the fact reported by one Canadian psychiatrist. He states that 40% of Alzheimer's cases are misdiagnosed! That's a real conversation stopper in the medical field! Very similar symptoms to those of this illness are sometimes due to a serious deficiency of Vitamin B12, or to a Vitamin E deficiency, hypochyroidism, cerebrovascular disease or a reaction to a drug.[37]

I have certainly known people diagnosed with Multiple Sclerosis (MS) who in fact suffered from a serious B12 deficiency. Again, symptoms of MS are similar to symptoms of a B12 shortage, so perhaps this Canadian psychiatrist's comments are correct.

If a member of your family has been diagnosed with Alzheimer's disease, dowse and ask if their illness has been correctly diagnosed. If you receive a 'No' answer, dowse and ask if they suffer from a vitamin B12 deficiency? Then ask if they suffer from a vitamin E deficiency? You can then ask if they suffer from Hypothyroidism?

A Finnish Study which involved 1,500 sufferers showed the presence of a high cholesterol level and high blood pressure problem tied to Alzheimer's. Dowse and ask if the sufferer in your family has a cholesterol or blood pressure problem? [47]

Is there a link between Alzheimer's disease and a diet which includes a regular intake of Trans Fats and Saturated Fats? A study 'Dietary Fats and the Risk of Incident Alzheimer's Disease' by Martha Clare Morris ScD *et al.*, involving 815 people, found strong statistical correlation between dietary intake of fats and the risk of Alzheimer's.

Dowse and ask the following questions:

1. Is there a link between intake of Trans Fats and Alzheimer's disease?
2. Do Trans Fats in the diet make you prone to Alzheimer's?
3. Do Omega 3 Oils in your diet help to prevent you developing Alzheimer's disease?

A study was reported in 'Archives of Neurology' which showed the intake of both Trans Fats and Saturated Fats promoted the development of Alzheimer's.[48] By dowsing, you will be able to establish which of the above facts will help to reduce symptoms of this distressing illness.

ANOREXIA – BULIMIA

There can be many reasons for young people to suffer from Anorexia or Bulimia. It's so easy when you are a teenager to over react to casual remarks about your weight or appearance and get it completely out of proportion.

The National Institute of Mental Health reports that eating disorders frequently occur with other mental disorders such as depression, anxiety disorders or substance abuse.[67]

As well as sufferers looking unflatteringly skinny, the induced regular vomiting can damage the oesophagus, and also enlarge certain glands. Anorexia can slow the heart rate and lower the blood pressure.

If a member of your family suffers from Anorexia or Bulimia, dowse and ask the following questions:

1. Is the regular vomiting damaging their oesophagus?
2. Is their blood pressure too low?
3. Is their heart rate affected by this illness?

If the sufferer has been starving her body of nutrition for some time then there is a very strong possibility that his or her body is very short of certain amino acids, minerals and vitamins, but the big problem is 'How do you get a determined teenager to take pills?' Well, the picture is not as black as it first appears. This is a case for 'Pendulum First-Aid'!

Sit down quietly and mentally cleanse your energy by bringing a beam of white light down through the crown of your head, through your body and into the ground. Then send a beam of this light through your pendulum to cleanse it. Now you can use the Pendulum Emergency Service to send the necessary supplements to the sufferer.

You can start by mentally asking the pendulum to please help to send the person everything her body requires for good health, following these steps: Swing the pendulum and ask it to please send the sufferer all the amino acids needed to bring them to the right level for good health and to please show you the 'Yes' sign when this work has been done.

Next, repeat the exercise but this time ask the pendulum to please top up the sufferer's body with the correct level of minerals, and again ask to be shown the sign when the job is complete.

Now ask the pendulum to please channel the necessary amount of vitamins to replace missing vitamins, and show you the sign when done.

After completing these three steps, you can dowse and ask if the sufferer's body has the correct level of minerals, vitamins and amino acids. This exercise can be carried out for all illnesses, so don't be afraid to experiment with your pendulum. It will work for you provided it has been cleansed and your energy is balanced. If you are in doubt about the state of your energies, you can ask a friend to dowse. If your friend discovers that your energies are not balanced, they can ask their pendulum to balance your energies. You are then ready to help the sick person.

Many Anorexia sufferers have been short of Zinc for some time, so ask the pendulum if the sufferer has Zinc deficiency. This can suppress appetite. Some sufferers also benefit from B6 and Serotonin but, as the pendulum has sent them all the minerals and vitamins they require, your work is done for the moment.

When the pendulum channels vitamins, minerals, amino acids or plants to a person, it is important to check a week later to ask if they require further supplies. This is particularly important in the case of Bulimia, as their vomiting will deplete the body's supply of everything necessary for good health.

It is a good idea to ask your pendulum to check if the 7 main chakras are correctly balanced as these are the power points of the body and, if any are out of balance, it affects health. If you receive confirmation that they are not all balanced, you can ask the pendulum to please balance them and show you the sign when they are balanced.

It is important to ask your pendulum to check if this person is either sleeping or working over Geopathic Stress (GS) from underground water or rock cracks, as this energy weakens the immune system and is the basic cause of many health problems. If your pendulum confirms the presence of this negative energy, then ask it to please remove the GS and balance the energy of the building.

ASTHMA

Asthma attacks are a nightmare for many mothers, as the number of young children who suffer from this upsetting illness is rising steadily. In the UK alone, there are several million sufferers.

The World Health Organization estimate 300 million people suffer from this illness and in 2005 it claimed the lives of 255,000 people. They forecast the death toll from Asthma will increase by 20% in the next ten years, unless a cure is found.[51]

Most of us take comfortable breathing for granted and never think about our 'in' breath or our 'out' breath, but for the many millions of Asthma sufferers in the world, it is a very different story. Asthma sufferers experience blocked airways, tight chest and difficulty breathing comfortably, often causing uncomfortable coughing and wheezing.

This chronic lung disease is a condition of the airways (the tiny tubes which carry air in and out of the lungs). Trouble occurs when the bronchial tubes and the trachea become inflamed, which causes the air passages in the lungs to narrow. Breathing becomes a real effort. Sufferers can experience many symptoms such as a blockage in their airflow and terrific tightness in their chest. There are several factors which trigger the illness and can cause this reaction of the airways becoming inflamed and occasionally blocked by mucus. Dowsing will help to find minerals and plants to give relief.

Dowse and ask if your Asthma attacks are caused by any of the following. If you receive a 'Yes' answer, then dowse each one separately. (1) Dairy products, (2) Food colouring, (3) Pollen, (4) Cat fur, (5) Moulds, or (6) Dust mites?

In addition, you can ask these questions:

1. Would my body benefit from taking a course of MSM organic sulphur? This mineral can help the body to form the protein structure so sufferers can often find relief.
2. Is my body short of B Vitamins? – these work by decreasing the inflammation in the lungs.
3. Ask your pendulum if B12 would improve the wheezing?
4. Would my body benefit from extra Vitamin C? – this vitamin is needed by asthma sufferers, as it helps the body to fight infection. It also reduces inflammation and is known to help increase the level of oxygen to the area.
5. Would a supplement of Pan D'Arco reduce the inflammation? This is a wonderful, well respected natural antibiotic used by many therapists to reduce inflammation.
6. Can the well-tried medicine from the ancient old tree Ginkgo Biloba help reduce the number of attacks?
7. Is your body short of Selenium?
8. Magnesium is known to decrease wheezing – ask your pendulum if your body is short of magnesium?
9. Ask if your Adrenal Gland is balanced?
10. Does Ephedra from Brazil dilate the bronchial tubes?

An old cure is to cover the chest with cabbage leaves nightly for three weeks. These act as a poultice and draw out inflammation. Dowse and ask if this remedy would help to reduce the asthma symptoms?

Natural cures are always the best way to treat any illness. An amazing natural treatment called Asthma and Bronchitis Herbal Formula is available from Regenerative Nutrition (*see index*). This treatment consists of liquorice root, slippery elm bark, and lobelia. Dowse and ask if this remedy would reduce the asthma symptoms? Also dowse and ask if it could reduce the number of asthma attacks?[2]

A supplement well worth trying is Propolis. This natural antioxidant comes from the bark of trees and tree buds and many sufferers have found that this simple supplement has helped to reduce symptoms. Propolis comes with good references – honey bees use Propolis to protect their hives from bacteria. It's also known to have been used by ancient Greeks, Romans and Egyptians 3,000 years ago, so it has certainly stood the test of time.[61]

A study reported on the Environmental Defence website states that during the 1996 Olympic Games when all downtown roads were closed to private cars, the number of hospitalised Asthma attacks were reduced by 20%. Does this prove that traffic pollution is linked to Asthma attacks?

Dowse and ask your pendulum if pollution from traffic can cause an Asthma attack? Ask if it is an irritant? You can phrase the question several different ways.[60] Here in the UK, 5.2 million people are receiving treatment and one in every ten children suffers from Asthma. This is an average of three pupils in each school classroom, so these figures give you an idea of the enormous scale of this illness. The UK has the highest prevalence of severe 'Wheeze' in children aged 13–14 years worldwide, so what is the cause? Every fifteen minutes a child is admitted to hospital in the UK suffering from this illness, so what is so different about Britain compared with Europe or other countries?[64] Certain exercises which teach deep abdominal breathing can relieve symptoms. Spiritual healing is also beneficial, as it enables the patient's body and mind to relax.

Probably the best alternative therapy to help teach controlled breathing is the popular Pilates. These courses are fun and you don't need to feel self conscious – everyone in the class is learning the correct way to breathe, as most of us do not get the maximum benefit from our breathing. If you feel awkward about joining a class, you can find a Pilates teacher to give 'one to one' coaching.

It can be money well spent as when you become aware of your breathing and learn how to control it (provided you've eliminated food from your diet which is causing an allergic reaction) you'll find your symptoms improve. Correct breathing will benefit your health and if you ask anyone who has attended a Pilates course, they will assure you that their health benefited and many of their painful back, shoulder or neck problems improved along with their general health.

Dowse and ask if your Asthma symptoms would be reduced by regularly doing Pilates breathing exercises?

Asthma and pregnancy

Can life in the womb decide whether or not a child will suffer from asthma? An interesting project at Aberdeen University on Asthmatic children found mothers who had eaten four apples a week during pregnancy were half as likely to have children who developed Asthma, compared to those who did not eat many apples during their pregnancy.

The project involved 2,000 mothers who were quizzed about their eating habits during pregnancy and then the child's health was checked five years later. This fact is worth considering if you are pregnant, as anything which stops a child from developing Asthma has got to be good news. Dowse and ask if eating four apples each week during pregnancy will benefit the health of the foetus?

Then dowse and ask if eating four apples each week during pregnancy will help to stop your child from developing Asthma? Perhaps the person who first quoted 'An apple a day keeps the doctor away' knew what he was talking about![72]

Asthma and dust mites

The Healthy Flooring Network issued the blunt message that fitted carpets are a prime culprit in the rise of Asthma cases. Dr Jill Warner, Senior Lecturer at Allergy and Immunology at the University of Southampton, reports that dust mites and their droppings trigger various allergies, including Asthma.

It is hard to believe the fact that many of us share our home with multi millions of mites, as there are up to 100,000 uninvited mites living in a square metre of carpet!

Dowse and ask the following questions:

1. Are there thousands of dust mites living in the carpets in my home?

2. Are my Asthma symptoms linked to the presence of dust mites?
3. Will the Asthma symptoms be reduced if carpets are removed?

The British have the highest number of carpets in their homes as over 90% of households have carpets, compared to 16% in France and 2% in Italy. Is it only a coincidence that Britain has the highest number of Asthma and Allergy sufferers in the world, or are dust mites one of the main causes of Asthma?[75]

ATHEROSCLEROSIS

Atherosclerosis is a hardening of the arteries caused by plaque forming on the inner walls of arteries which causes them to become congested, thereby reducing the level of blood which is able to pass through.

The arteries affected by this problem can be in several different areas, including the heart, where arteries affected by this problem can cause angina or coronary thrombosis. Arteries in the brain can also be affected by a build up of plaque, which can be the cause of a stroke. Another area which can be victim to Atherosclerosis is the kidneys.

It's clear that this plaque can create real problems in several areas of the body. Dowse and ask if a supplement of Chromium will slow down the progression of the illness? Then dowse and ask the pendulum if your body is short of Chromium.

Serrapeptase? It is an enzyme which is particularly good at removing plaque. Dowse and ask if a supplement of Serrapeptase would be beneficial?

Sometimes sufferers are deficient in certain amino acids, so dowse and ask if your body is deficient in the amino acid Taurine? Then dowse and ask if your body is deficient in the amino acid L'Carnitine?

Vitamin E is known to do a good job of unclogging plaque, so dowse and ask if a supplement of vitamin E would be beneficial. Then ask if it would assist with unclogging the plaque?

Beta-Carotene is an anti-oxidant which plays an important role in attacking free radicals in the body, and is beneficial to many Atherosclorosis sufferers. Dowse and ask if your body would benefit from a supplement of Beta Carotene. Dowse and ask your pendulum if a supplement of Beta-Carotene would be beneficial to your health?

Myrrh is an anti inflammatory, antibiotic and antifungal gum resin from this tree grown in Africa and India. Dowse and ask if a supplement of Myrrh would benefit your health?

Some good news is that Guinness and Stout are reported to be beneficial for this illness, so sit down and enjoy a glass of this much favoured drink!

ATHELETE'S FOOT

You are left in no doubt when you suffer from Athlete's Foot. This exasperating fungal infection causes the most aggravating itch between the toes, particularly if you wear socks of man-made material which do not absorb perspiration. It thrives on warm and damp places so when the central heating is on during winter and your feet feel hot, or when the weather is warm in summer and the heat makes your feet sweaty, the ideal conditions are created and the fungus is happy. Symptoms of its presence include scaly or cracked skin between the toes. So how do you declare war on this virus?

This fungus does not like fresh air and sunshine, as it thrives when the feet sweat. In some cases it can spread to the toe nails. It is very easy for this fungus to move from one person to another, as it lurks in damp places like swimming pools or sports club locker and changing rooms.

There are many products available in the pharmacists, but sufferers assure me the most efficient weapon when fighting this virus is a diluted solution of grapefruit seed extract. Anti fungal cream is available from any pharmacist.

Tea tree oil, Colloidal silver and Grapefruit seed extract are all natural treatments to cure infection and are known to kill harmful bacteria. Dowse and ask if bathing the infected area with a solution of Grapefruit seed extract will kill the virus? Then ask the same question of Tea Tree Oil and Colloidal Silver.

AUTISM

Autism is a neurological disorder which affects the sensory motor and neurological functions, and is the third most common childhood development in the US.

Confirmation that autism is becoming a much more common illness comes from the Federal Department of Education in California who report an increase of 1700% over the past ten years. This is a pretty staggering figure and brings home the full extent of the increase of autism.[54]

It can strike any family for no obvious reason and the most frightening fact is that this problem is escalating at a horrific rate. In the UK, figures bring home the severity of the problem. It's estimated that one in every 175 school age children is thought to have a form of autism. In the USA, diagnosed cases of Autism are increasing by 20% each year.

So what is the cause of the dramatic increase in this distressing illness? An unreleased report from the US Centers of Disease Control states that exposure to more than 62.5 micrograms of Mercury within the first three months of life is a cause of this illness.[36] For more information on this subject see www. autismfraud.com

One's first reaction is 'Where on earth can so many babies be exposed to this heavy metal, since the illness affects children in many cities and villages?' The answer is vaccination! Most babies receive more than 62.5 micrograms of mercury through the paediatric vaccines in the first few weeks of life, but hopefully things are changing. Thimerosal, used as a preservative in vaccine, contains mercury so the finger is pointing firmly at Thimerosal.[36]

A symptom of this illness which is first diagnosed in early childhood is a noticeable withdrawal into themselves and detachment from surroundings.

A research survey commissioned by Generation Research which involved 17,000 boys in the 14–17 age group showed alarming results. Vaccinated boys were 155% more likely to develop neurological disorders than unvaccinated boys and 224% more likely to have ADHD. These figures increased with age; in the 11–17 age group, boys were 317% more likely to have ADHD and 112% more likely to have Autism. Dowsing will confirm if these worrying figures are roughly correct.

Dowse and ask the following questions:

1. Does the child's body have excess tartic acid?
2. Is the child short of magnesium?
3. Is the child's body short of Vitamin B6 or B12?
4. Is the fungus Candida present in the child's body?
5. Is the child's body short of Iron?
6. Are the levels of the child's stomach acids out of balance?
7. Would the child benefit from a supplement of DMG (Dimethylglycine)?

You can use the pendulum to balance any shortages.

Symptoms – Is your child 'Low Active' – switched off – not hungry? Dowse and ask if he would benefit from a supplement of Absorbic acid.

Is your child Hyperactive with ADHD type symptoms? Dowse and ask if a supplement of fish oil would reduce symptoms.

Is your child aggressive and always hungry? Dowse and ask if he would benefit from a course of calcium carbonate.

There appears to be a strong link between some cases of autism and routine childhood vaccines containing Thimerosal. Some children have been found to have very high levels of mercury in their blood. Is it a coincidence that Thimerosal is a mercury based preservative used in vaccines? Dowse and ask if your child's autism is linked to excess mercury in the blood? Also ask if the illness is linked to Thimerosal? You can ask your pendulum if it is possible for an experienced dowser to remove the vibration of mercury from the blood with the pendulum.

Medical News Today report 4,800 parents are involved in the US Federal Claims Court. These folks are all parents of autistic children and many of them blame Thimerosal for this dreadful plight.

In 2003, after a three year long investigation, the US Government Reform Committee concluded that Thimerosal is likely related to the autism epidemic which could possibly have been prevented.[26]

There's been a big cloud hanging over Thimerosal for well over a decade. Back in 1982, the FDA proposed regulations to remove this drug from certain products. In July 1999 the FDA took further action and requested that manufacturers remove Thimerosal from vaccines, as some children were receiving unsafe levels of mercury as high as 30 times the minimum acceptable level.[49]

So is this drug in any way linked to the fact that one in every five children in the US, and many in other countries, suffer from learning difficulties?

Thimerosal is a mercury-containing organic compound, so it makes sense to avoid any product containing mercury when possible as this heavy metal is known to be the second most toxic element on Earth (Plutonium being the first).[49] Please get dowsing and ask a variety of questions on vaccinations containing mercury which could be linked to Autism.

Will we ever be able to return those children from their distant world back to our world? There is research being done on sub-atomic particles such as electrons which are actually able to communicate with each other literally billions of miles away in a split second – the message moves faster than light. This is a whole new world of medicine, but progress is being made, so dowse and ask if it will ever be possible to remove damaged particles in the brain caused by the vaccine which have been responsible for the damage to health. I believe that if we can remove the damaged particle and reprogram it then the message will get to suppliers of this vaccine. It sounds far fetched, but dowse and ask if my thoughts are correct on this subject?

Doctors keep telling us 'Breast is Best' but what about the chemicals like Thimerosal and various heavy metals which are in the mother's milk or in her blood? Dowse and ask if Autism can be caused by the presence of chemicals or heavy metals in the mother's milk? Then ask if this illness can be caused by chemicals or heavy metals present in the mother's blood?

There is a lot of research being carried out on the use of Enzymes to treat many illnesses. Dowse and ask if a supplement of certain Enzymes would reduce the symptoms. You could also dowse and ask if the Enzymes should be combined with a Vitamin B supplement?

Also dowse and ask if Food Intolerance is linked to the Autism? If you receive a 'Yes' answer, dowse and ask if the child is allergic to cow's milk or dairy produce.

Another possible problem can be a Candida overgrowth in the child's gut. This is another common symptom, so dowse and ask if Candida overgrowth is present in the child's gut?

Have you ever considered a course of Chelation therapy for your child? This modern day therapy removes heavy metals from the body. Removing heavy metals such as arsenic, mercury, aluminium and lead from the nervous system can show a great improvement in symptoms of autism. Dowse and ask if your child would benefit from Chelation therapy?

Next, dowse and ask if your child has heavy metals in their system. If you receive a 'Yes' answer, you can then dowse to establish which heavy metal is in their system. You can then ask the pendulum if it is able to remove the vibration of the metal from the child's body? If you receive a 'Yes' sign, cleanse the pendulum and then hold it and ask it to please remove the vibration of the heavy metal from the child.

There are so many possible causes of this escalating problem, so where do you start in this minefield? I think the most important question to ask when you dowse for treatments for autism is 'Is my child sleeping over Geopathic Stress (GS) energy?' This energy will weaken the child's immune system so that his body is unable to fight off health problems. If you receive a 'Yes' answer to the presence of GS, then ask your pendulum to please clear the Geopathic Stress energy from your home and show you the 'Yes' sign when the job is complete. GS is powerful negative energy which comes from underground water deep under the foundation of the building, and is often present in many homes where illness has occurred.

A question which puzzles doctors is 'Why are there four times as many autistic boys as girls?' One reason could be that, whereas the female hormone estrogen decreases Thimerosal's toxic effect, the male hormone Testesterone greatly increases its toxicity. Dowse and ask if these facts are correct.

Recently published research has found that children suffering from Autism have much lower than normal levels of Glutathione, Homocysteine and other amino acids in their body.[38] As these amino acids do an important job of protecting the body against heavy metals including mercury, it is important to maintain the correct levels of amino acids. Dowse and ask:

1. Is the child's body short of the amino acid Glutathione?
2. Is the child's body short of the amino acid Homocysteine?
3. Ask if they are short of any other amino acids? If you receive a 'Yes' answer you can either purchase amino acids from a health shop or use the pendulum to top up the level in their body. If you use the pendulum to do this work, the level needs to be checked regularly, and please remember to cleanse your pendulum.

It is so important to keep searching for a cure to bring these children back from their world into our world.

BABIES – LABOUR

It's all very well telling women that labour is a natural process and to some women it is a wonderful experience, but to others it is a living nightmare. So much depends on the size and position of the baby, as well as the mother's anatomy. However, there are things we can do to make this process easier.

Dowse to ask if Selenium would help avoid a difficult labour? Also check if the body is short of manganese?

I recommend attending the National Childbirth Trust classes. You will be able to learn how to help your body relax to allow contractions to be most effective, and the importance of breathing to control pain. This breathing stands you in good stead when you go to the dentist or any other unpleasant experience!

BACK PAIN

Back pain is a common complaint and most of us suffer from this tiring ache at some time in our lives. When it's constant, it totally disrupts your lifestyle and as nothing is to be seen, you don't get any sympathy!

Dowsing is an excellent tool to diagnose the root of the pain or stiffness. The pendulum will confirm if the pain is caused by the pelvis being out of alignment or a nerve being trapped. It may simply be wear and tear from years of doing work which strained the back, or perhaps an old sports injury.

Muscular and joint pains respond well to certain plants and minerals, so get the pendulum out and ask if any of the following supplements will improve the problem and relieve symptoms: (1) Glutamine, (2) Boswellia, (3) Chondroiton, (4) Zinc/Copper or (5) Manganese?

Can a massage or chiropractor treatment release the build up of crystals? Also ask if a supplement of Serrapeptase will reduce scar tissue.

If your back muscles regularly go into spasm to protect a damaged area, dowse and ask if regular walking will strengthen the muscles and help to resolve the problem.

BALDNESS

Today there are all sorts of treatments for baldness and, as they say, 'bald men are very virile.' Perhaps it's a good thing to be bald!

Dowse and ask if the body is short of tin. If you get a positive answer, you can use the pendulum to channel the vibration of tin to the person.

Now dowse and ask your pendulum if the person's body is short of selenium. Will a supplement of Selenium encourage hair growth? Ask if a supplement of this antioxidant will benefit their health? Dowse and ask if your body is short of essential fatty acids, sulphur, lysine, iron or Vitamin B12?

BELLS PALSY

Symptoms of Bells Palsy are easily recognised as the facial muscles of the sufferer weaken or can become paralysed due to an upset in a cranial nerve.

Bells Palsy can affect either side of the face and can occur where the body's immune system is low. Fortunately the paralysis only affects the face and not other parts of the body. Although this is a distressing illness, the symptoms usually improve within a short period, with the exception of a very small percent of sufferers. It is not contagious, so will not affect other members of the family.

Dowse and ask the following:

1. Is Bells Palsy caused by a Calcium deficiency?
2. Will a supplement of Echinacea improve the condition?
3. Is the patient's body short of Copper?
4. Will a supplement of Mistletoe improve the condition?

Please consider a course of Healing, as this problem responds well to healing energy.

BLOOD CLOTTING

A stroke is a very debilitating illness which can rob the patient of speech or power of movement. To offer help and create awareness of this illness, the UK Stoke Foundation was formed. www. ukstrokeforum.org

A stroke is caused by the blood supply not reaching the brain. This can be caused by a small clot of blood. Less common is a fatal stroke, which is caused when a blood vessel bursts and blood flows to the brain. Dowse the following topics:

1. If a member of your family has suffered a stroke, please dowse and ask if they have been sleeping or working over a Geopathic Stress line? If you receive a 'Yes' answer then ask the pendulum to please neutralise this energy.
2. Ask your pendulum if a supplement of Serrapeptase would help to clear the plaque? This enzyme removes clots and scar tissue.
3. As blood clots create a real health risk, it's worth considering all treatment no matter how off putting it sounds! Dowse and ask if Hirudin from leeches would prevent blood clots? Hirudin is known to dissolve clots after they have been formed.
4. Dowse if Antistatin from Mexican leech would reduce blood clotting? Ask your pendulum if Tick Anticoagulant Peptide (TAP) would remove clots? Dowse and ask if the herb Knotted Figwort will dissolve the clots?
5. Guarana is known to thin the blood, so ask if Guarana would be beneficial?
6. Sarsaparilla cleanses the blood so ask your pendulum if it will help your blood problem.
7. Cat's Claw works wonders on many health problems and is known to thin blood clots so dowse and ask if will help your blood problem.
8. Horse Chestnut is also known to thin the blood and break up clots.

Sarsaparilla, Guarana, Horse Chestnut and Cat's Claw are all available from local health shops.

Omega 3 essential fatty acid can reduce platelet aggregation which can lead to blood clots and strokes,[40] so ensuring your blood has sufficient essential fatty acids is doing your body a big favour. Dowse and ask if your body is short of Omega 3? Then dowse and ask if Omega 3 is beneficial to your blood? This oil is free from side effects.

High blood pressure is a very common problem and simply means that there is a high blood pressure in the arteries. It's considered to be 'high' when it registers 140/90. The next time someone tells you they have high blood pressure, you'll know that it is simply the pressure with which our blood pumps the blood in the body into our arteries.[26] It is really important for the blood pressure to be maintained at the correct level as, if it is too high or too low, then illness can follow. So what can we do to reduce high blood pressure, a very common problem?

The Adrenal Gland plays a very important part in checking pressure, so dowse and ask if this gland is balanced. Then ask your pendulum if the Pineal Gland is balanced, as these glands are often out of balance. Dowse and ask the following questions:

1. Does your body have a deficiency of the amino acids L'Arginine? Then ask if it is deficient in Taurine.
2. Is your body low in certain minerals? If 'Yes' then ask – would your health benefit from a supplement of (a) Magnesium (b) Potassium (c) Germanium or (d) Melatonin?
3. Would a supplement of Hawthorn reduce symptoms?
4. Cat's Claw is known to help sufferers, so dowse and ask if a supplement would lower blood pressure?
5. Ask if your body has too high a level of Cadmium? Cleanse your pendulum and ask it to please remove the excess Cadmium.

An old fashioned cure is to rub olive oil on the kidneys. As these old wives tales often work very well, dowse and ask if this treatment would be beneficial?

Use the pendulum to ask if the Ions are balanced. When they are correctly balanced, the Negative should be more than the Positive.

As well as dowsing for suitable supplements, you can dowse to find the cause of the High Blood Pressure.

Dowse and ask if it is caused by tension in your life?

Ask if it is caused by an age related narrowing of arteries?

Ask if it is caused by an illness in the kidneys or other area?

By establishing any shortage of amino acids or minerals, you will be able to rectify the deficiency and so improve your symptoms.

Do you suffer from High Blood Pressure? Well, it's not all bad news. Doctors at Germany's University Hospital of Cologne have found that research results show a small amount of dark chocolate eaten daily, as well as brightening up your day, can reduce blood pressure.

Research results have shown that in the group who ate a small amount of dark chocolate two hours after dinner over a 4 month period, their systolic blood pressure dropped by almost three points and their diastolic pressure dropped by two points.[34] These results were published in the Journal of the American Medical Association.

For the past 2,000 years Noni fruit has been used in China and India to treat blood pressure as this fruit contains a phytonutrient which dilates previously constricted blood vessels, allowing blood pressure to become normal. Dowse and ask if the Noni fruit will reduce your blood pressure problem? Noni is available from Regenerative Nutrition and is a natural product.[79]

- Horse Chestnut is an anti haemorrhagic – it breaks up clots.
- Blood Root (Indian plant) prevents excess bleeding.
- Guarana thins blood, so it separates clots and helps to prevent thrombosis.
- Beetroot will help to build new blood.
- Echinacea helps the body cope with blood poisoning.
- Vitamin K stops haemorrhages.

Your pendulum will confirm which treatment will be beneficial to your blood. If there is a serious problem with your blood, you need to visit a haematologist who is a specialist in this field.

A high percentage of everything we put on our skin travels into our blood stream, and if you are a woman who uses make-up on a daily basis, you could be absorbing as much as 5lbs of chemicals into your body each year, and some of these chemicals are definitely not 'people friendly'.

Parabens contained in many skin and hair products can be dangerous, as traces of this group have been found in breast tumour samples. It's astonishing how many cosmetics and hair products contain this group of chemicals which includes methylparaben, ethylparaben, propylparaben, butylparaben and isobutylparaben.

Sodium lauryl sulphate, as well as being absorbed into the blood, can cause skin irritation and is known to irritate the eyes.

The National Institute of Occupational Safety and Health report nearly 900 of the chemicals used in cosmetics are toxic.[43] You can dowse the products you use.

Dowse and ask if the shampoo you use contains any toxic harmful chemicals? Ask the pendulum if your cosmetics contain harmful toxic chemicals? Ask each jar or bottle separately. Now ask if any of the chemicals in your beauty products soak through into your bloodstream?

Propylene glycal is used to maintain moisture and can cause contact Dermatitis. It's also known to be linked to depression of the central nervous system. If you would like to know more about chemicals found in cosmetics, and also a list of UK stockists of chemical free cosmetics, contact the Woman's Environmental Network www.wen.org.uk[44]

The Campaign for Safe Cosmetics points the finger at the following chemicals: **Mercury** – found in certain makes of eye drops and also in some brands of deodorant and ointments. **Formaldehyde** and **Toluene** – found in some brands of nail products. **Petroleum distillates** – found in some makes of mascara, perfume, foundation, lipsticks and lip balm. **Coaltar** – found in certain dandruff shampoo and hair dyes. **Dibutyl Phthalate** – found in some brands of nail polish, perfume and hair spray. **Lead acetate** – found in some hair dyes and cleaners.

The Environmental Working Group's Skin Deep website lists troublesome products and advises us that Grecian Formula Hair dye contains lead acetate. Today, all lead is removed from household paint and also from gasoline, due to its danger. Lead acetate is banned in Canada, although not in the US.

Dowse the following questions:

1. Do my eye drops contain mercury?
2. Does my deodorant contain mercury?

3. Does my deodorant contain aluminium?
4. Does my mascara or perfume contain petroleum distillates?
5. Does my lipstick or lip balm contain petroleum distillates?
6. Does my nail polish contain Dibutyl Phthalate?
7. Does my nail polish contain formaldehyde?
8. Does my hair colour contain lead acetate?

Please take the presence of chemicals in your body very seriously. Toxic exposure can be transmitted to future generations as a 'Second Genetic Code'[81] and can program sections of our children's DNA. Remember that any chemicals present in cosmetics and household products can soak into your blood stream, so dowse and check before purchasing any new brand.[45]

We are constantly exposed to chemicals in the food we eat, the air we breathe and the water we drink, and if that is not bad enough, chemicals are constantly being added to our atmosphere from industry.

It is hard to imagine but there are roughly 80,000 industrial chemicals in commercial use in the USA alone.[53] Many of these chemicals are not 'people friendly' and are linked to damage to the immune system, cancer and reproductive problems. Our blood has a lot more problems to face than the blood of any previous generation.

The Campaign for Safe Cosmetics is a coalition of health and environmental organisations who have for several years been putting pressure on cosmetic companies and personal care product manufacturers to phase out chemicals linked to birth defects, cancer and other health problems.

In 2007, the EU introduced a policy requiring all companies that either produce or use chemicals to collect extensive data on possible health risks of these chemicals. Unfortunately things are different in the US as under US law, the FDA does not test, review or approve cosmetics and personal care products before they go on sale and only a few colour additives and other substances are banned.

This means that companies can put virtually anything they choose into their cosmetics, which is one very good reason to dowse each product you use. Checking if they contain any harmful ingredients and establishing whether or not they can soak into your bloodstream is very important.[78]

I have talked about the chemical research that has revealed chemicals in our bodies, but what can we do to get rid of these chemicals? It is almost impossible to get rid of chemicals in the blood without assistance. There are herbs that can help to detox and alternative treatments which specialise in this work. The main thing is to be aware of this invisible hazard which is constantly in our midst, and take evasive action.

Start by reading the list of ingredients on all of your household cleaning products. The 'Bad Guys' which, when possible, should be avoided are: Alcohol, Ammonia, Formaldehyde, Phenol, Perchlore Benzenes, Propellants Glycols, Hydrochloric Acid and Ethanol.

In personal care products try to avoid Sodium Laureth Sulphate, Glycerin, Alcohol, Propylene-Glycol and Parabens. Those of you who are old enough to remember ingredients granny used for cleaning and first aid will know that they were very effective, completely harmless and the big benefits were that they were both cheap and natural. It is time to say good-bye to window and mirror cleaning sprays, polish, worktop and sink cleaners, and go back to basics. Your granny or great granny will be 'up there' smiling down on you and nodding that at last you've learned sense!

Try discovering the joys of Baking Soda sold as Bicarbonate of Soda and sometimes nicknamed Soda Bic. This multi use powder is available in most food stores and is inexpensive. It is very mildly abrasive so great for cleaning worktops or the top of the cooker, and added bonuses are that it has whitening properties and it deodorises.

Another 'old wive's friend' is good old vinegar. Vinegar is multi purpose; it makes a good job of cleaning mirrors and windows, and as it's acidic, it is a powerful tool to attack germs and remove grease. There are many housewives who will be pleased to tell you of their many uses for this inexpensive liquid.

If you have an unwelcome growth of mildew or mould in your home, an excellent way to get rid of this unwanted visitor is to purchase Borax. It has been around for a very long time and has been well tried and tested by women for decades and still remains a popular anti fungal.

Today, statistically, we may live longer than our predecessors but what about our quality of life? This extension is paid for dearly by modern chemicals and drugs in daily use, and the waxed fruit and the vegetables containing chemicals in our diet. It is time to take stock and dowse for the presence of unhealthy chemicals in your life.

BONE INJURIES

Olive Oil is a very useful addition to your First Aid Kit. It's a remedy used all through the ages. As a child, I can remember my mother treating injuries using warm olive oil which came in a bottle wrapped in straw. The use of this oil goes much further back in history than my childhood; the Bible tells of the Good Samaritan pouring oil on the man's wounds.

Olive Oil is a natural remedy free from side effects and beneficial for strains and rheumatic type aches. This cold pressed oil is beneficial in healing bone damage, so whether you suffer from a cracked or broken bone, or a bone marrow problem, dowse and ask if this oil will benefit your injury? Ask your pendulum if it will speed up the healing process?

Propolis is a natural healer, so it's a good supplement to help regenerate bone mass after you've suffered a bone injury. This great healer is an antioxidant and free from side effects.[61]

BURNS

There are three separate categories of burns: the first degree burn involves the outer layer of the skin. The second degree burn is when the outer and second layer of skin have been burned. The third degree burn is by far the most serious and involves all layers of skin.

You can dowse and ask if the burn is first degree – if the answer is No then call medical assistance, as second and third degree burns needs urgent treatment.

Dowse and ask if Calendula will help to heal the minor burn, then dowse and ask if Colloidal silver will keep it clear of infection? You can use your pendulum to channel Colloidal silver to the burns victim and you will probably be amazed at how quickly the wound repairs and heals.

CANCER

There are many very different causes of cancer and many different treatments and possible cures, so this is where dowsing becomes an invaluable tool. It enables you to find the most suitable treatment, and also the cause of the cancer.

Certain cases of cancer can be caused by a shortage of Melatonin in the body, so dowse and ask the following questions:

1. Is my body short of Melatonin?
2. Will my body benefit from a course of Melatonin?
3. Can Melatonin help my body to fight the cancer?

Childhood cancer is on the increase and a question often asked is 'Can high level of exposure to a television set influence the melatonin level in the child's body'? We all get an uneasy feeling about our children spending too much time watching television and playing video games. Perhaps our fears are justified. A research study in Italy found children who abstained from watching TV and video games and computers had a much higher level of Melatonin in their urine sample at the end of the one week period when they did not have access to a TV set, than the samples of their urine taken before the week's trial started.[17]

So if exposure to the TV screen is reducing the level of Melatonin in their body, is this linked to the increase in childhood cancer? It also raises the questions 'Is the EMF (electromagnetic field) energy from the TV screen the cause of the reduced level of Melatonin, or is this reduction linked to light from the screen? It's an interesting question and it's important to find the correct answer, as many cancer patients have a shortage of Melatonin.

Dowse and ask the pendulum the following questions:

1. Does several hours' exposure to EMF's from a television reduce melatonin in the child's body?
2. Does exposure to light from the TV screen for several hours reduce melatonin in a child's body?

Surely if the children's body level of Melatonin is lowered by TV viewing then adults will also be affected! Dowse and ask if the Melatonin level in adults is lowered by regularly viewing TV? Could this be one of the reasons for the steady increase in cancer cases?

B17, also known as Amygdalin & Latrile, is known to help fight most cancers and can be purchased without difficulty. Ask your pendulum if a supplement of Amygdalin will reduce the tumour?

If you have dowsed and the pendulum has confirmed that B17 would be beneficial then have a look at the Anti Cancer information website: http://www.anticancerinfo.co.uk. It offers valuable information on B17 to sufferers.[27]

There are many tried and tested natural methods of treating various cancers, and one which makes a lot of sense is altering the energy of the tumour. Raymond Grace in his book '*The Future is Yours, Do Something about It*' teaches us how to use the pendulum to scramble the frequency of the tumour and to reprogram the tumour to a healthy frequency. This method is well worth considering as it's a simple exercise and the benefits could be enormous.

Cervical Cancer

Cervical cancer is the second leading cause of death in women in the 15 to 44 year age group and every day 40 women in Europe die of this illness.

Dowse and ask if this form of cancer can be caused by the human Papilloma virus?[50]

50

One school of thought suggests cancer is caused by the presence of a Flat Worm in the body, so dowse and ask if there is a flat worm infestation in your body? If you receive a Yes answer then ask if it is part of the cause of the cancer? There is medication available to get rid of any infestation.

Cancer seems to strike when the immune system is low and one thing most cancer sufferers have in common is that they either sleep or work over Geopathic Stress, which weakens their immune system. Research in Europe has confirmed this fact, so dowse and ask if you are sleeping over a Geopathic Stress energy line.

Scientists have for many years been looking in the most unexpected areas for cures for this dreadful illness and their search has included many ingredients from trees, plants, flowers, Australian coral, Caribbean Squid, and venom from Asian Pit Viper and Copperhead Viper snakes and the Israeli scorpions. Yes, some of these sources sound pretty far-fetched, but research has found some amazing success stories.

In the venom from the Copperhead Viper, the chemical Contortrostatin has been isolated and found to have the ability to put tumors to sleep by choking off their ability to feed and grow. Malignant gliomas (*tumour of the Neuroglia*) are a form of cancer not often curable, but it's Snake Venom to the rescue! Research at the Dept. of Neuro-surgery at the University of Southern California has shown that the ingredient Disintegrin Contortrostatin from the venom has the ability to inhibit the growth of the tumour and an added benefit is that it has no neurotoxic side effects. Dowse and ask if this treatment will benefit any tumour? More information is available from the LeadDiscovery website.[3]

Another snake venom used in the treatment of cancer is the venom from the Asian Pit Viper, which is known to inhibit the spread of Melanoma cells. Dowse and ask if the venom from this snake would inhibit the spread of Melanoma cells?

One fascinating treatment for Breast, Lung, Colon and Prostate Cancer is Cryptophycins, from the 3 million year old Blue Green Algae. Research results suggest the Algae can treat tumours which are immune to other drugs. Research at Lily Research Laboratories showed this to be a promising new class of anti tumour agent.[4] Dowse and ask if this treatment would reduce your tumour? If your pendulum confirms that the patient would benefit from this treatment, you can use your pendulum to send the vibration of any of the algae, snake or scorpion venom to help them.

A report in the Decatur Daily News tells us that Dr Harold Sontheimer and his team at the University of Alabama have shown in their research that the chemical compounds from the Giant Israeli Scorpion's venom could successfully kill cancerous cells in the brain. Not only that, it could perform this feat without harming healthy cells.[5] This venom is reported to bind cells and stop the spread of tumours.

With such an assortment of treatment available to channel with your pendulum, dowse and ask if the venom from the Israeli scorpion will reduce your tumour? The BBC News reported on 30th July 2006 that research has found that Scorpion Venom attacks tumours, so gradually awareness is spreading of the natural cures.[9]

The Caribbean Squid is another source of treatment – Ecteinascidin 734 has been isolated and found to be successful in treating breast cancer and melanoma cells. Pre-clinical trials show the ET-734 is active against a range of tumour types in animals including breast, colon, ovarian, lung, melanoma and several sarcoma. Dowse and ask if Ecteinascidin 743 will reduce your tumour? If you'd like further information, have a look at the Marine Biotech website.[6]

Many therapists agree that one of the best cures for cancer seems to be the natural herb Pau D'Arco (also called Lapacho) from the inner bark of the Taheebo Tree, grown in South America. This treatment has been used successfully by Indio tribes of the region for many centuries, so it is well tried and tested. The ancient Incas and Aztecs are reported to have recognised the healing powers of this tree, and modern science is now accepting the great medicinal powers of this wonderful tree and bringing it into its fold.[7]

Dowse and ask if Pau D'Arco will reduce your tumour. This herb is available in a tea.

The Madagascan Periwinkle – It's hard to believe when looking at this dainty and very pretty little pink plant that it could possibly be a successful treatment for certain cancers. This amazing plant, only found in tropical forests of Madagascar in the East African coast, has given us two cancer fighting medicines: Vinblastine, which is used in the treatment of Childhood Leukaemia and Vincristine which is now used to treat patients suffering from Hodgkin's disease.[8]

Dowse and ask your pendulum if a course of medicine from the Madagascan Periwinkle will reduce your cancer?

Cancer Research in 1988 at Columbia University showed that an active ingredient in Propolis could slow or completely stop the growth of several different types of cancer. Propolis is an anti-oxidant, anti-bacterial supplement from tree bark and tree buds, which seems able to raise the body's natural resistance to infection by stimulating the immune system.[61]

Cranberry juice has been recognised for several years as a successful treatment for prostate problems, and can also destroy the cause of ulcers, but Cranberry has lots of other benefits which are being discovered.

Researchers at Cornell University showed that it's something of a wonder juice as it killed bad cells. Other studies have shown that in lung tumours, colon and leukaemia, the cells died because the Cranberry juice inhibited growth.[68] Dowse and ask if several glasses of Cranberry juice each day will kill the cancerous cells in your body?

Then ask your pendulum if Cranberry juice can reduce the number of cancerous cells in certain cancers. Will it inhibit growth of all cancerous cells?

Cancer can be found in many areas of the body and as everyone's body is different, the reaction to different treatment can vary. Please don't worry about being confused by the number of possible treatments I mention in this chapter. You will be able to dowse and ask which is most suitable for your particular cancer.

Are organic tomatoes an excellent tool to fight cancer? The New Scientist reported results of a ten year study at the University of

California, Davis, which found these tomatoes contained considerably higher level of the flavonoids quercetin and kaempferal; 79% and 97% respectively. Flavenoids have been recognised for some time by scientists as an antioxidant, and linked to reducing rates of some forms of cancer and cardiovascular disease.[69]

Dowse and ask if organic tomatoes in the diet can sometimes help to prevent cancer? Ask if organic tomatoes would reduce your cancer?

Breast cancer

Patrick Holford of the Institute of Optimum Nutrition says we must explore every avenue to cure Breast cancer as already one in every eight women in the UK alone will develop it.[28] In other words, a woman in every other family and several women in every road and every office will develop this form of cancer.

When you think about it on this scale you will realise how important it is. Do dowse to try and find tools to fight this killer illness.

Research at the University of California in Los Angeles showed Omega 3 has the ability to ward off cancer by helping to maintain healthy breast tissue, and so prevent breast cancer.

Another study showed this dietary supplement of Omega 3 produced fewer quantities of a carcinogen associated with colon cancer, which provides even more confirmation that a supplement of Omega 3 is a way to better health.[41]

Bone cancer

Yet another product linked to cancer is fluoride. Over one hundred leading national and international cancer prevention scientists and representatives of consumer and environmental organisations have endorsed the Cancer Prevention Coalition's campaign opposing fluoride in drinking water. Their concern is due to research results that show bone cancer in young men is sometimes linked to fluoride. If anyone in your family is suffering from bone cancer, please dowse and ask your pendulum the following questions:

1. Can bone cancer be caused by fluoride in your drinking water, toothpaste or from amalgam fillings?
2. Can fluoride in the body cause any form of cancer?
3. Does fluoride in the water soak through your skin to the blood?

Fluoride is in 60% of US drinking water and 2% of Europe's drinking water. If you live in a home which has fluoride in the water it means that every time you have a bath or shower your skin absorbs a high percentage of this chemical. The skin is the body's largest organ. If it absorbs a lot of fluoride into the blood then could your health be at risk?

Dr Sam Epstein Professor Emeritus of Environmental and Occupational Medicine at the University of Illinois and Chairman of the Cancer Coalition supports the opposition to fluoride in the UK.[12]

There are so many foods, environmental effects, cooking utensils etc. blamed for the increase in cases of cancer, so being able to dowse enables you to eliminate those which could damage your immune system and leave it unfit to fight cancer.

Greenpeace UK report findings from Russian research which showed that laboratory rats fed on genetically modified potatoes developed cancer. While rats are different from us humans, anything that causes rats to develop cancer deserves attention and should ring a loud warning bell.

These research results from the Institute of Nutrition of the Russian Academy of Medical Sciences has been suppressed for eight years, but a court battle fought by environmental groups succeeded in releasing the data for public information. The report showed that rats fed on GM potatoes developed tumours and suffered serious damage to their liver, kidneys and large intestines. The GM Russet Burbank potato fed to the rats contained the antibiotic marker gene, which is a sobering piece of information. Not surprisingly, Greenpeace stated that these potatoes must not be used to feed people.[13] Perhaps it's just as well we do not know exactly what we are eating in many of our meals!

Dowse and ask the following:

1. Can regularly eating GM Russet Burbank potatoes cause cancer?
2. Can the antibiotic marker gene in the potato cause cancer?
3. Can the antibiotic marker gene in the potato cause health problems?

We have so little information about the various additives, genes etc. added to our food that it is almost becoming a necessity to dowse certain foods before purchasing them! Perhaps in years to come we will all be wandering down the aisles in the local supermarket with our pendulum swinging over foods!

Certain researchers firmly believe that cancer is linked to a shortage in the body of silver, so dowse and ask if a silver deficiency is linked to cancer? The body only needs a minute trace of this mineral but if it is missing, then health can be affected.

Mouth and throat cancer

Researchers in the UK are working on a treatment to reduce the risk of infection to sufferers of this dreadful illness, and are busy testing the effects of raw honey from the Manuka bushes, which is believed to have powerful healing, anti-infection and anti-inflammatory properties.

These researchers expect the honey to promote healing and protect against bacterial infection. Honey has been used for many centuries to heal open wounds. Dowse and ask if Manuka honey will benefit anyone you know who suffers from this form of cancer.[21]

Brain cancer

Why are more and more brain tumours being diagnosed today than ever before? This form of cancer is becoming more common and figures in the USA have increased by 25%. What is causing the unexplained rise in this form of cancer?[56]

Scientists know that exposure to mobile phone radiation can cause human brain cells to shrink, so is mobile phone use a cause of brain cancer? Is this the reason Lloyds of London refuse to insure mobile phone manufacturers against damage to user's health?

Dowse and ask if regular mobile phone use can be a cause of brain tumours? Also, dowse and ask if the sufferer is sleeping over Geopathic Stress?

Chemicals and cancer

Is the widespread use of chemicals linked to the enormous increase in cancer sufferers? A study reported in the British Medical Journal estimated that 75% of cancer cases are caused by environmental and lifestyle factors. Even worse is a report from Columbia University School of Public Health which suggests 95% of cancer cases are caused by environment and diet. These figures seem pretty frighteningly high until you realise that somewhere between 400 and 800 chemicals are stored in most people's bodies.

Dowse and ask if harmful chemicals are stored in the body of most people in the Western world? The sort of chemicals and toxins in the environment which I am talking about are:

1. Phthalates which can disrupt the body's endocrine glands. As they play an important part in good health, damage to these glands is very bad news.
2. Pesticides; The Environmental Protection Agency (EPA) reports 90% of fungicides, 60% of herbicides and 30% of insecticides are known.
3. Carcinogens. Alarmingly, between 50% and 95% of pesticide residue have been found in US Food. This fact confirms it is wise to dowse your food for the presence of harmful toxins, heavy metals and carcinogens.
4. Heavy Metals including Arsenic, Aluminium, Cadmium, Lead and Mercury are all present in our atmosphere and their presence is often linked to neurological diseases and cancer.

In the US alone there are vast amounts of chemicals produced each year, and when you add those figures from Europe and other countries, the scale of the toxins in the atmosphere is alarming.

Dr Mercola reports the following figures:

1. Roughly 77,000 chemicals are produced in North America.
2. Over, 3,000 are added to our food supply.
3. More than 10,000 chemical solvents, emulsifiers and pre-servatives are used in food processing.
4. Around 1,000 new chemicals are introduced each year into our atmosphere.[30]

So where do these chemicals go? They end up in rivers, lakes and oceans, and some seep through the ground to underground water supplies, which is the reason much of our underground water supplies are contaminated.

Arsenic and cancer

We know that arsenic is very harmful to our health so most of us avoid it at all costs, but it is hard to avoid this heavy metal when it's hiding in your chicken dinner. So what on earth am I talking about?

The Union of Concerned Scientists report that many chicken products sold in the USA contain this carcinogen. No, it isn't some dramatic news flash to sell more newspapers; the facts are included in a new report by the Institute for Agriculture and Trade Policy. The investigators found arsenic in half of the 155 samples from supermarkets and in all, 90 samples from fast food restaurants.

Arsenic is legally fed to roughly 70% of broiler chickens to kill parasites and promote growth.[20] Perhaps we'd be better eating the parasites, as at least they are not carcinogens! I assume the level fed to chickens is not above the legal level but it could create a health problem by adding to the arsenic already in our body from the environment. Eating this chicken is bad news and to add to the problem, the poor chickens who have digested the arsenic then give the environment their 'droppings' which must be contaminated with arsenic.

The Food Trading Standards Office has advised me that in the UK, the legal limit of arsenic added to chicken feed varies depending on the diet.

Dowse and ask if the chicken you are having for dinner contain above the legal limit of arsenic? Dowse and ask if Arsenic is a carcinogen?

Childhood cancer and chemicals

We often ask why the number of cases of childhood cancer is on a steady increase. One answer could be the fact that a large number of children's bath products contain a cancer causing petrochemical.

It's bad enough that this ingredient is in baby shampoo and bubble bath but the evil fact is that in some cases, it's more than twice the US Food and Drug Administration's recommended maximum level. Many of these brands are on sale in Europe, UK and other countries.

The cancer causing petrochemical is called 1,4-Dioxane and is a clear cut animal carcinogen. It's a suspected cause of both cancer and birth defects.

1. Dowse and ask if the shampoo you use on your child's hair contains this chemical?
2. Is this chemical a carcinogen?
3. Is this chemical in your child's bubble bath?

When we purchase shampoo or other cosmetics, we assume the product has been checked for health effects before being marketed but unfortunately this does not happen. The FDA does not review or regulate cosmetic products for safety, and ironically this enormous department does not have the legal authority to intervene on our behalf.[58]

This is another time when you'll be glad you learned to dowse. You can check each product for harmful chemicals before purchasing products for children.

Skin cancer

Skin Cancer is not only common in areas of Australia and the US where radiation from the sun is very powerful, but according to figures from the World Health Organization (WHO), 3 million people each year develop non-melanoma skin cancer, and 132,000 develop melanoma skin cancer. Another figure reported by WHO which surprises most of us is that one in every five people in America will develop skin cancer in their lifetime, and one in every three cancers diagnosed is a skin cancer.[55]

Basal Cell carcinomas are by far the most common skin cancers and fortunately these are slow growing cancers and very seldom travel to other areas of the body.

Squamous Cell carcinomas also seldom spread. The most serious skin cancer is Melanoma, as this cancer can spread to other parts of the body and is often difficult to cure. Skin Cancer can often respond well to a supplement of vitamin B17, so dowse and ask if a course of this vitamin would help to heal your skin cancer?

Skin cancer is reported in many cases to be successfully cured with the use of urine therapy. Simply soak a pad in fresh urine and leave on the skin cancer for 24 hours before changing the pad. Yes, I agree it sounds an unusual and anti social treatment, but if it cures the cancer then it has to be good news. When you stop and think about it you will realise that urine is 100% sterile when it leaves the body so cannot pass on any infection to the wound.

We are all regularly warned of the importance of using a sun screen on our skin if we are going to be exposed to strong sunlight to avoid melanoma of the skin, which is a particularly unpleasant experience, but is this correct advice? Back in 2003 Dr Mercola warned us that sun-blocks can actually cause skin cancer by blocking the skin's absorption of ultra violet radiation and so blocking the much needed production of Vitamin D in your skin. Studies have shown that vitamin D can prevent roughly 77% of all cancers, where as most sunscreen lotions contain cancer causing chemicals![73] This is an interesting topic and dowsing will tell you if it is more beneficial to block the sun's rays or to allow them to penetrate your skin. Ask your pendulum if certain brands of sunscreen contain cancer causing chemicals?

Research studies on the incidence of melanoma in Scandinavia and the USA found a strong association between the introduction of FM Radio Broadcasting and an increase in the number of sufferers of skin cancer.

The research results suggest it is exposure to the radio frequency which weakens the body's cell repair mechanism due to the body resonating electromagnetic fields. This seems to amplify the carcinogenic effect of cell damage caused by UV radiation.[18]

It is an interesting report, so let's dowse and ask the following questions.

1. Is FM Radio Broadcasting at full body frequency linked to an increase in melanoma cases? Dowse and ask if the research results are correct?
2. Can melanoma be caused by UV rays from the sun?
3. Can melanoma be caused by a combination of exposure to UV rays and rays from FM Radio stations?[20]

Prostate cancer

Results of a research study newly released at the American Society of Clinical Oncology's Annual Meeting displayed hope for prostate cancer sufferers. This study showed that when taken for 30 days, Flaxseed seemed to slow the growth of these tumours.

In the study, 161 men due to undergo a prostatectomy were separated into four groups. Duke University reports that those men in the two groups taking 30 grams of flaxseed powder had by far the slowest rate of growth of their tumour – the cells grew 30% to 40% slower. Flaxseed contains Omega 3 fatty acids so is an excellent aid to good health.[29]

Lycopene is a powerful anti oxidant which is known to be a good pal to the prostate. This is found in tomatoes, tomato sauce and also apricots, guava and melons. Green Tea is also well known as an excellent anti-oxidant which can help to remove prostate cancer, and I must mention Selenium which is found in Brazil nuts and is an excellent antioxidant.

Chemotherapy

Glutamine is thought to repair the gut lining after chemotherapy treatment, and sufferers report that taken three times each day it can reduce the unpleasant side effects of the treatment.

Astragulus taken before the chemotherapy treatment is thought to protect the liver. If you or a member of your family is going to receive chemotherapy treatment, then dowse and ask your pendulum if they would benefit from taking a course of Glutamine or Astrogulus?

Liver cancer

Why do more men than women develop liver cancer? The human body produces a protein called Interleukin-6 (IL6) which is linked to liver cancer. As well as women's body producing less of this protein, research at the University of California, San Diego, showed women's production of estrogen controls the amount of this protein IL6 they can produce. Men produce higher levels of IL6 as they do not have estrogen to control the levels.

Dowse and ask if the protein IL6 is linked to some cases of liver cancer in men? Ask your pendulum if this is the reason more men than women develop liver cancer? There are more cases of bladder cancer in men than women, so dowse and ask if the protein IL6 is linked to certain cases of bladder cancer in men? Dowse and ask if giving men an estrogen type compound would reduce the cases of liver cancer?[39]

We hear stories of so many possible cures for cancer and one may suit one person and another cure works for someone else. However, if I am ever unfortunate enough to develop this disease, my first port of call will be the local shop to purchase a carton of Bicarbonate of Soda!

How often do you hear folks say that the simplest cure is often the best, and how often do you find that the cure or the answer has been looking you in the face and you don't see it? Well perhaps that's what is happening in cancer research. Are researchers looking for a cure in complex genes, when the answer is in our kitchen larder?

The oncologist Italian Doctor Tullio Simoncini has been very successfully treating cancer patients with the powerful anti-fungal Bicarbonate of Soda. I am somewhat biased in favour of this treatment as I belong to the generation who used 'Soda Bic' for many first-aid treatments.

Dr Simoncini's research has shown that cancer is linked to a common fungus Candida Albicans, and reports that we should never underestimate the power of Fungi as this is a force which science does not yet fully understand.

Of all the human parasite species, he explains that Candida Albicans fungus is by far the most powerful, and emerges as the sole candidate for tumour proliferation as it can be carried through the blood and lymph glands. Bicarbonate of Soda is able to attack fungi across the spectrum of all its forms, and this is the only way it can be irradicated. It is very important to strengthen the patient's immune system to help fight this determined organism.

Dowse and ask the following questions:

1. Can Cancer be caused by a fungus?
2. Is Cancer ever caused by Candida Albicans fungi?
3. Can a regular high dose supplement of Bicarbonate of Soda kill the Candida Albicans fungi?
4. Can your pendulum channel the vibration of Bicarbonate of Soda to the fungus?
5. How many times per day? Per week? How many weeks?

If your pendulum confirms that the cancer is caused by a fungi, dowse and ask if any of the following anti yeast will help to weaken the fungi?

MSM, Wormwood, Mathake and Pan D'Arco as these are all known as anti-parasite pills and reliable, powerful weapons in the fight against parasites.

If your pendulum confirms that Bicarbonate of Soda, which is an inexpensive white power, could attack your tumour then perhaps you'd like to find out more about the treatment from the book

'*Cancer is a Fungus: A Revolution in the Therapy of Tumours*' by Dr Tullio Simoncini, available from http://www.cancerfungus. com.[70]

Dr Simoncini assures us that Bicarbonate of Soda is a very simple treatment which causes almost no side effects apart from thirst and a feeling of weakness.

CANDIDA ALBICANS

Candida is caused by a powerful, yeast-like fungus which can infect mucus membranes. Removal of this parasite can be very successful with certain minerals and plants. So how does this' organism get into the body? Many folks blame a course of anti-biotics, so dowse and ask if this is the root cause of your Candida? This unwelcome yeast organism needs to be ejected from your body, and MSM is often the answer, as MSM reduces the yeast infection and helps to eliminate the harmful micro organisms.

Barley Grass Juice Powder is rich in chlorophyll and is anti-bacterial. It is a good source of easily digestible protein which is a gentle detox and is very rich in antioxidants.[1]

Wormwood (*Artemisia Absinthium*) is a little known plant which offers a reliable treatment for Candida, as this herb has an excellent anti-parasite action which removes an invasion of parasitic fungus. The anti-parasite action of Wormwood has been known and used for thousands of years to eliminate a range of worms and parasites including Candida.[74]

Dowse and ask if a supplement of Wormwood will be beneficial.

1. Will Wormwood reduce the parasites in my body?
2. Can Wormwood kill Candida parasites?
3. Will a beneficial effect be felt within 14 days?

Dowse and ask if your body will benefit from a supplement of any of the following medication: (1) Boron, (2) Manganese, (3) Mathake (*kills yeast*), (4) Pau D'Arco (*anti yeast*), (5) Lapacho, (6) Cinnamon (*anti yeast*), (7) Acidophilus, (8) Molybdenum, (9)

Chromium, (10) Aloe Vera, (11) Germanium (*increases oxygen*), (12) Oil of oregano (*contains natural fungicide – 4 drops*).

CARPEL TUNNEL

Carpel Tunnel Syndrome is an extremely painful problem which can affect the hand and wrist. It's caused when the carpel tunnel which protects the median nerve becomes swollen and inflamed. It can also be due to Dupuytren's contractions in the hands which create a thickening of some fibrous tissue or gristle in the palms. This pulls the tendons of one or more of the fingers, resulting in the fingers being bent over.

An operation is often necessary to undo the damage, but things are looking brighter for sufferers of Carpel Tunnel. The enzyme Serrapeptase is able to help sufferers. This amazing enzyme linked to the silk worm is able to eat scar tissue around tendons and also remove any blood clots or inflammation. The big bonus is that it does not appear to have side effects.

I have been taking a supplement of this enzyme for a couple of months and a damaged ligament with lots of scar tissue has now become pain free. A back injury has also been resolved, so I am totally sold on this little known enzyme.

Dowse and ask the following questions:

1. Is my body short of Copper?
2. Is my body short of Vitamin B6 or B12?
3. Would a supplement of Vitamin E relieve the problem?
4. Would a supplement of MSM Sulphur relieve symptoms?
5. Would a supplement of the enzyme Serrapeptase help to reduce the problem?
6. Will a supplement of Echinacea strengthen the immune system?
7. Is my body deficient in Iodine?
8. Are you sleeping over Geopathic Stress?

It is well worth dowsing to ask if any of the above items will reduce this problem. It's important to avoid an operation on the hand as it can make a life a little complicated while the wound is healing.

COLITIS

Ulcerated Colitis is an auto immune illness caused by abnormal activity of the immune system in the intestines, leading to chronic inflammation of the colon. I have treated many sufferers of this distressing illness over the years and found that symptoms of this inflammation usually improved dramatically when the patient takes a course of Chromium tablets and Brewers Yeast. Even those with a Yeast intolerance still seemed to benefit from Brewers yeast, so dowse the following questions.

1. Will a supplement of Brewers Yeast help my body to fight the Colitis?
2. Will a supplement of Brewers yeast reduce the symptoms?
3. Will a supplement of Chromium reduce the symptoms of Colitis? Now ask if your body is short of Chromium?
4. Will a supplement of Glutathione improve the symptoms?
5. Will Butoryic Acid reduce symptoms?
6. Will a supplement of Echinacea strengthen my immune system?
7. Is my body deficient in iodine?

Ask your pendulum if you are sleeping or working over Geopathic Stress too, as this energy is often present in the homes of sufferers of Colitis.

CONJUNCTIVITIS

Conjunctivitis is recognised by the Pink or Red inflammation around the eyes. It is often itchy and sticky and can be passed on, so it should be treated and never ignored.

Bathing with Eyebright reduces inflammation and makes the eye more comfortable. I understand that beta carotene and zinc are both beneficial and 2000 mg of Vitamin C is often helpful, so dowse and ask if a course of Vitamin C will help to heal the conjunctivitis? Then dowse and ask if bathing with a solution of Eyebright will help to reduce the problem?

Dowse and ask if a supplement of beta carotene will improve the condition and then ask if Zinc will heal the eye problem. This mineral has an excellent reputation for healing wounds and infections.

CONSTIPATION

Constipation is a common bowel problem caused when the stools become solid and the causes are many and varied. Some folks suffer severely when they go on holiday or away staying with friends, while others have suffered since childhood.

This problem can be linked to diet – too much dairy produce might be the cause. Another common cause can be a shortage of magnesium oxide in the diet. The plant Golden Seal is known to soften the stools, so dowse and ask if any of the following are linked to your constipation problem.

1. Is the problem caused by emotional stress?
2. Is it linked to a shortage of magnesium in the body?
3. Does dairy produce cause my constipation?
4. Will a supplement of any of the following items improve the problem? Golden Seal, Magnesium oxide at bedtime, Ispaghula, MSM.

CRAMP

Cramp is an extremely painful experience and can occur at the most inconvenient time. It's caused by a contraction of muscles and is most common in the legs, feet and stomach. Muscle cramp in the limbs can be caused by lack of salt or a deficiency of magnesium. It can often occur after excess exercise, particularly if it causes you to perspire as sweating causes the body to lose salt.

You can treat this form of cramp either with heat or an ice pack. I find a hot water bottle works wonders – the heat relaxes the muscles and gives comfort.

Nocturnal cramp in the calves of your leg or in your foot is a nightmare. The pain is intense and you frantically try to get out of bed in order to get your foot on the ground to allow the blood flow that relieves the pain. The medics say these night cramps are a 'niggle' which comes with old age, but it can also affect any age group. A really powerful attack of cramp can leave a reminder the next day. Your leg can feel bruised and painful. So what can you do to deter this night time disturbance and avoid attacks at other times?

Muscle cramp can sometimes be a symptom of Hypothyroidism, so test if your body is short of iodine. Paint a small amount of iodine tincture about the size of a 5 pence piece on the inside of your wrist or thigh when you go to bed. In the morning if the bright colour of the Iodine is still on your skin then your body is not short of iodine, but if the colour has faded then you are deficient. (Some folks paint the iodine on the soles of their feet as it is less conspicuous.)

Dowsing will help to find the root cause of the cramp, so ask your pendulum the following questions:

1. Is the cramp caused by a mineral deficiency?
2. Is it caused by a thyroid problem?
3. Is the cramp caused by lack of salt in my body?
4. Is it caused by a Magnesium deficiency?
5. Will Homeopathic Ferr Phos supplement reduce cramp?
6. Will a supplement of Magnesium reduce the cramp attacks?
7. Will a supplement of Magnesium/Calcium reduce the attacks?
8. Is my body short of Iodine?
9. Am I sleeping over Geopathic Stress energy?

All of the above minerals can be purchased from a health shop and once the cramp attacks have ceased, it's important to dowse regularly to establish if your body has the correct level of these minerals. Your body's needs change and you may no longer require these supplements.

If you are sleeping over Geopathic Stress, sit down quietly and ask your pendulum to please remove the Geopathic Stress energy from your home and to show you the 'Yes' sign when it has been done. Hopefully, after going through these steps, you can say good bye to Cramp!

CRAVING FOR CERTAIN FOOD

An unexplained craving for chocolate is often your body telling you it is short of B vitamins while a craving for sweet things like biscuits and cakes is often a sign that your body is short of Chromium. This uncontrollable urgency to eat biscuits which can make you frantically search cupboards in the hope of finding a packet is usually under control after you add a supplement of Chromium to your diet. Chromium is available from all health shops.

Dowse and ask your pendulum if your body is short of Chromium? Also dowse and check if Lycopodium (Nelson's Tissues) would solve the problem. Dowse and ask if L'Glutamine will stop the craving symptoms.

CROHN'S DISEASE

Crohn's Disease is an ongoing illness caused by serious inflammation of the digestive tract. The disease can cause the sufferer to experience acute abdominal pains, diarrhoea and rectal bleeding. Dowse and ask if your body would benefit from any of the following supplements? (1) Zinc, (2) Vitamin B, (3) Folic acid or (4) Glutathione.

Ask your pendulum if your illness is linked to the measles virus. If you receive a 'Yes,' you can ask the pendulum to remove the vibration of the measles virus.

Ask your pendulum if there is an infestation of the flat worm parasite in your body. If you receive confirmation then you'll find a remedy by a visit to the health shop.

Dowse and ask if a supplement of Omega 3 would help ease your symptoms. Fish oil is recognised as beneficial to the illness.

And finally, it is important to check that there is no Geopathic Stress in your home as this will aggravate your health problem.

CYSTIC FIBROSIS

Cystic Fibrosis is caused by a fault in the genes which affects the lungs and causes them to become vulnerable to infection. Salt and water in the lungs become dried out. This dreadful affliction is an inherited chronic illness which affects the lungs and digestive system. The defective gene and its protein product cause the child's body to produce a sticky mucus which can clog the lungs and obstruct the pancreas.[46]

Dowse and ask if any of the following will improve some of the symptoms:

1. Would a supplement of Silica improve symptoms?
2. Would a supplement of the enzyme Serrapeptase reduce the mucus in their lungs?
3. Would a supplement of Hawthorn be beneficial?
4. Ask your pendulum if Coltar would relieve the symptoms.
5. Would a supplement of Malt be beneficial?
6. Ask if a supplement of Creosote Bush would help to relieve symptoms.
7. Ask if Geopathic Stress is present in the home?

Although this distressing illness is considered incurable by the medical profession, some of the above suggestions will help to relieve symptoms and regular Healing sessions will be beneficial.

CYSTITIS

Cystitis is a very painful and annoying inflammation of the bladder, usually caused by an infection, which affects millions of women each year. Fortunately, the infection usually only lasts a short time and does not normally cause any long term problems.

70

This infection is caused by bacteria which travels from the skin and grows in the bladder. Symptoms can include a stinging or burning sensation when passing urine and an urge to urinate when you know very well your bladder is empty.

Some sufferers experience lower back pain, lower abdominal pain or blood in their urine. If you experience any of these symptoms, it's time to start dowsing to check if you have Cystitis?

1. Ask your pendulum if your bladder problem is caused by Cystitis?
2. Ask if drinking plenty of water will clear the infection?
3. Will adding a teaspoonful of Bicarbonate of Soda in drinking water clear the infection? Bicarbonate of Soda helps to balance the acid/alkaline level.
4. Will a teaspoonful of Colloidal Silver three times each day remove the infection?

Dowse and ask if any of the following supplements would help to reduce the symptoms: (1) Nettle Tea, (2) Cranberry Juice, (3) Blueberry Juice or (4) Bearberry juice. Bearberry Juice clears urinary tract infections and Cats Claw helps the body to fight the infection.

Drinking plenty of water to flush the system helps to clear the infection and use unperfumed soap when possible.

DEMENTIA

Symptoms of Dementia include a loss of the person's intellectual abilities (such as their memory capacity). The symptoms can be so severe that they completely disrupt the sufferer's social and occupational functioning. Sufferers can experience disorientation, inability to concentrate and an unreliable memory. Additionally, this illness plays havoc with their language, motor and spatial functions.

In the past 25 years there has been an astronomical 300% increase in the number of cases of brain disease such as Dementia, Alzheimer's and brain tumours. This increase is only in countries where Aspartame the artificial sweetener is used. Dowse and ask the following questions:

1. Is Aspartame in the diet linked to any brain illnesses?
2. Do any of the contents of Aspartame damage health?
3. Is Dementia linked to Aspartame in the diet?

There are so many possible avenues to explore and as research has shown, this artificial sweetener affects children's behaviour; it's therefore quite possible that it is linked to brain illnesses. Dowse and ask if your health would benefit by excluding this artificial sweetener from your diet?

In recent years, research has shown that aluminium from cookware and deodorants can damage health. Aluminium free deodorants are now on sale in most stores. Dowse and ask if this heavy metal can be a cause of Dementia? Channel Ascorbic Acid to the brain to repair impaired glucose transporters. Dowse and ask if a supplement of Gingko Biloba would be beneficial. Ask if a supplement of any of the following would help to reduce symptoms: (1) Taurine amino acid, (2) Zinc (*improves memory*), (3) Folic acid, (4) B12 or (5) Vit C.

DEPRESSION

Depression is a mental disorder which is affecting more and more people, causing lack of interest, lack of motivation and lack of self worth. It can cause the sufferer to have dark moods and thoughts, experience tiredness and lack of appetite and (as if that wasn't enough) many sufferers have a disrupted sleep pattern.

In some cases sufferers of severe depression feel life is not worth living. In fact, the World Health Organization figures show 850,000 deaths a year occur from this illness. Worldwide there are roughly 121 million sufferers of this illness.[52] This is an illness which needs more recognition urgently.

So what is the cause of such a common health problem? Many folks are short of money or become unemployed, but is it more than that? Is our diet linked to this modern day illness?

If anyone in your family suffers from Depression, there are certain basic questions to ask in order to help establish a cause and a cure. Often the cause can be exposure to chemicals, shortage of minerals, or sleeping over Geopathic Stress energy. Dowsing will help to find the answers to this health problem.

What causes Depression? While there are many different sources of Depression, it can often be caused by bereavement, loss of employment or abuse of drugs. Another group of sufferers are unfortunate enough to have it in their family history.

Research has shown that patients who suffer depression have a smaller Hippocampus than normal, which can create a problem – this tiny part of the human brain is vital to the storage of memories, but the main problem with a smaller hippocampus is that it has fewer Serotonin receptors. As this is an important neurotransmitter, having the correct level in the body is vital to good health.[25]

Dowse and ask if the patient's hippocampus is smaller than the normal size? If the answer is 'Yes', then you know the correct level of Serotonin is not getting through.

Now dowse and ask the patient's body is short of the neurotransmitter Serotonin? An excellent source of information on Serotonin is Oliver James' book 'Britain on the Couch' which explains in great detail the work of Serotonin and its beneficial effect on health.

Serotonin is often at a low level when the sufferer feels suicidal or suffers panic attacks.

Dowse and ask the following questions:

1. Is the sufferer's body short of Serotonin?
2. Is Serotonin deficiency often linked to Depression?
3. Will a supplement of Serotonin reduce the symptoms of Depression?
4. Does a shortage of Serotonin link to most psychiatric illnesses?

Also shown in research is the fact that Cortisol, which is a stress hormone involved in the working of the hippocampus, is produced in excess in patients suffering from depression.

Dowse and ask if the patient's body has the wrong level of the hormone Cortisol in their body? If you receive a 'Yes' answer, you can ask if this problem can be resolved. Then ask if an experienced dowser can balance the level of this hormone with a pendulum?

Tryptophan lifts depression, and is helpful for over wrought or agitated sufferers. 75% of patients have a depressed thyroid function, so dowse and ask if the person suffers from this problem. Many sufferers find relief from Tryptophan but it's not on sale in the UK. It is available on the internet. You can also use the pendulum to channel it to the sufferer; simply ask the pendulum to please channel the correct amount of this amino acid to the patient and to show you the 'Yes' sign when the task is complete.

A low production of the thyroid hormone can cause chronic depression so check. Also check the level of vanadium? Dowse and ask if the patient has the correct level of Vanadium? If you receive a 'No' answer, ask the pendulum to please correct the balance.

Ask the pendulum if the Hypothalamus is balanced? Then ask if the pituitary glands are balanced. If they are out of balance, you can use the pendulum to correct the balance. When that exercise is finished, it is time to balance the pineal gland – again, use the pendulum to check the balance.

Patients suffering from Mental Health problems can sometimes find the root of the problem is a parasite infestation and when this has been removed, the problem is lifted. Frank Strick, Director of the Research Institute for Infectious Mental Illness in California states that patients suffering from mental illness are likely to have a much higher rate of parasite infestation than the general population.

A fascinating fact is that a single mature tapeworm can lay one million eggs a day, which is a pretty impressive feat. Roundworms, which are known to affect roughly 25% of the world's population, lay 200,000 eggs each day. Confirmation that worm infestation is a common occurrence comes from The World Health Organisation, who report that over two billion

people are infested with worms. If any friends or members of
your family suffer from Depression, Candida, loss of sex drive
or lack of motivation, then dowse and ask if they have a worm
infestation?[33]

Amino Acid Methionine and Amino Acid Phenylethalmine,
when taken with vitamins, can lift depression quickly.

Dowse and ask the following questions:

1. Can a supplement of Folic Acid alter the body's Histamine
   level?
2. St John's Wort is a gentle treatment, would it be beneficial?
3. Will Tyrosine (an anti depressant) be helpful for apathy,
   lethargy and listlessness?
4. Glutamine can help to lift Depression. Ask if a supplement
   will be beneficial?
5. Dowse and ask if the negative and positive ions in the body
   are balanced? They can be disrupted by exposure to electromagnetic fields.
6. Dowse and ask if the frequency of the brain is out of balance? If you receive a 'Yes' answer, ask if it is possible to
   use the pendulum to balance the frequency of the brain?
   This is not as daft as it sounds – remember, we are all
   made of energy!

Depression comes in three types:

- Major Depressive Disorder.
- Dysthymia, which is a less severe depression but has long
  lasting symptoms.
- Manic Depressive illness, known as Bipolar disorder, is
  the most serious form of this illness and can affect social
  behaviour.

Depression is a much more common illness that most of us
realise as many sufferers don't say much about this problem.
Back in 2001, the World Health Organisation reported that
Depression (not Bipolar) was the leading cause of years lived
with a disability among men and women worldwide. That's a

very sobering thought and makes you aware of the scale of this health problem.[25]

If you would like more information on this subject visit the MedicineNet.com website. They have information on many illnesses. Please note that if you suffer from Depression, it's important to get another person to dowse for answers on your behalf as the negative energy in your body linked to this illness can affect the answers given by the pendulum.

Omega 3 essential fatty acid is needed to enable the body to function properly. A deficiency is linked to depression, mood swings and other mental health problems.[42] Dowse and ask if your body is short of Omega 3? Then dowse and ask if your depression would be improved by a supplement of Omega 3 oil?

There are many causes of Depression so it is worth exploring every avenue to find a cause and a cure.

DIABETES

The illness Diabetes is a metabolic disorder causing either high blood glucose or insufficient Insulin. The hormone Insulin is produced by the pancreas and if the workings of this important organ are disrupted, trouble follows. Insulin has the important job of controlling the glucose level in the blood and if there is a breakdown in this department, glucose may stay in the bloodstream. Hypoglycemia is diagnosed.

Deep trunk bending several times each morning will improve symptoms as the action of your tummy pressing on the pancreas stimulates it. This exercise is described in *Helping and Healing by Thomas Haberle*. It is a simple cure but those are often the best.[22]

There are two very separate categories of this health problem: Type 1 and Type 2. Those who suffer from the latter have a pancreas which is not producing any insulin, so insulin injections are essential.

Type 2 Diabetes is said by the medical profession to be incurable, but is this really true?

Dowse and ask if Type 2 Diabetes is a curable illness? Also ask your pendulum the question 'Is *my* Diabetes Type 2 curable?' One sufferer cured his advanced Type 2 Diabetes by removing all the modern day manmade fats from his diet.[10]

Dowse and ask your pendulum if eating man made fats is linked to Diabetes type 2? It is an interesting thought and if it is correct, it is an easy way to remove the symptoms of this illness.

How do you know when you suffer from this illness? The most common symptoms are unexplained thirst, hunger and tiredness. Another symptom is an increase in trips to the 'loo'.

Dowse the following topics:

1. Bearberry Tea is thought to remove excess sugar in the blood. Dowse and ask if a supplement would be beneficial?
2. Aloe Vera is known to relieve symptoms in some sufferers and garlic is beneficial. Dowse and ask if a supplement of either will improve symptoms?
3. An allergy to Cow protein can initiate Diabetes, so dowse and ask if a reaction to cow's milk triggered this illness?
4. Many sufferers are short of Chromium, which is known to enhance the function of insulin and therefore plays an important part in health. Dowse and ask if your body is short of Chromium. Then ask if a Chromium supplement would be beneficial (available from all health shops).
5. Dowse and ask if your body is short of MSM, B12 or Zinc, as these all play an important part in reducing symptoms of this illness.
6. Ask your pendulum if a supplement of any of the following would be beneficial to your health.
7. Vanadium controls insulin. Is your body short of Vanadium?
8. Would a supplement of Pfaffia be beneficial? This plant from the rain forest is a great tonic for many illnesses.
9. Ask your pendulum if a supplement of any of the following would improve symptoms? Periwinkle flower, brewers

yeast or lapacho. You can use the pendulum to send your body whichever of these are required. The exercise should be repeated in a week's time.

10. Dowse and ask your pendulum to please tell you if the chakras are balanced? The Solar Plexus chakra is often out of balance in people suffering from this illness. If your pendulum confirms that any of your chakras are out of balance, ask it to please balance them and show you the 'Yes' sign when done.

Next, you can experiment with a good old fashioned cure recommended by a monk! Remove the hard stalk from a cabbage leaf, place the leaf on your lower abdomen each night and leave it there to do its work while you sleep. Not very good for romance but if it relieves your symptoms, it's been worth the inconvenience! The cabbage leaf has amazing healing qualities and can act like a poultice to remove poison.

Is your body short of the hormone Gastrin? Check if the body is making a sufficient amount of the hormone Gastrin. One sign of a shortage is wind and flatulence. Your pendulum will confirm if there is a shortage of this hormone.

Back nearly a century ago, this was an almost unheard of illness, with only 2 persons in every 100,000 suffered this disease. Today, 16,000 persons out of every 100,000 are sufferers. It is now the third leading cause of death in the US. So what's different in our lifestyle today that could have caused this gigantic increase?

The World Health Organisation's figures paint a depressing picture. They report that roughly 180 million people worldwide suffer from Diabetes and deaths from this illness are around a million each year. The most depressing fact quoted is that they expect the number of deaths to increase by 50% in the next 10 years and predict that Diabetes deaths in the upper middle income countries will increase by 80% between now and 2015.[76] That's one good reason to dowse to find the cause and a cure.

One expert suggests that in the 20's, folks ate plenty of sweets and cakes and cooked with lard and dripping, whereas today we cook with oils. Is the use of cooking oils in our diets in some way linked to Diabetes?[16]

It is certainly an interesting thought and one which we can dowse. Ask your pendulum if the increase in the number of Diabetes sufferers is linked to the use of ingredients in certain cooking oils?

You can phrase the question differently and perhaps ask your pendulum if some cooking oils or fats disturb the balance of the pancreas? You could also ask the pendulum if cooking with lard or dripping is healthier than cooking with certain oils.

Childhood Diabetes is on the increase too – is it aggravated by watching more than two hours of television each day? Does it affect the blood sugar level in children suffering from Diabetes?

At the University of Oslo, researchers lead by Hanna D. Margeirsdottir M.D. showed that in a group of 538 13-year-old children, blood/sugar levels rose higher with each hour of television or computer viewing. The implications of these results are serious as so many children with this illness spend several hours each day using their computer and playing computer games, as well as watching television programmes. Are these children damaging their health?[23] Dowse and ask if these results are correct? Ask your pendulum if viewing television for several hours each day will raise blood/sugar level?

This morning as I was typing this page, I received a clear message in my head that Juniper Berries are an excellent treatment for Diabetes. I telephoned a dowser friend and asked her to ask her pendulum if Juniper Berry was a beneficial treatment for this illness. Her pendulum's reaction was amusing – it was so enthusiastic about the question that it swung in an enormous circle confirming the message I had received. For further confirmation I typed Juniper berry on the screen to do a Google search and lo and behold, here was more confirmation.

Oil of Juniper, which is an oil used in aromatherapy, would be an ideal treatment as a high percentage of everything that goes onto our skin goes through to the blood. I also found a product advertised by MicroNutra Health called Diamaxol, which claims to be 98.2% effective for Type 2 diabetes and 60% for Type 1. Of the 98.2% who benefited, 93.2% of them said their blood sugar level was now normal.[24] That's a pretty impressive track record, so dowse and ask your pendulum if this product would be beneficial? It is nice to think that one's symptoms can be regulated quickly with the aid of a box of pills.

Dowse and ask if a course of Diamoxal will help to balance the blood sugar level? Also ask if regular massage with Oil of Juniper would be beneficial?

I hope that among the possible treatments I have mentioned you will find one to reduce your symptoms.

DRUG AND ALCOHOL ADDICTION

Perhaps Drug or Alcohol addicts will think I am mad when I say this but, by taking the Alternative route, they may very well find it easier to kick the habit. Read on to find the simple cures!

If a Cocaine addict really wants to give up the habit, a useful tool to help is Emotional Freedom Technique (EFT). Tapping on important energy lines with your fingertips can give amazing results. Dowse and ask if a course of EFT's tapping would reduce cravings?

Now dowse and ask if the level of Prolactin in the body is out of balance? If you receive a 'Yes' answer, ask the pendulum to please balance the level of Prolactin as this will help to resolve the problem.

It's time to talk about Dowsing the advantages of a supplement of Ibogaine. Could this medication from a plant grown in Africa reduce the addiction? Ibogaine is derived from the root of an African plant the Tabernanthe Iboga, which appears to have the natural ability to treat both drug and alcohol addiction. It has been thoroughly researched over a period of years by Dr Deborah Mash, Professor of Neurology and Molecular and Cellular Pharmacology at the University of Miami. She reports that a trial involving 230 addicts produced utterly amazing results when long term heroin addicts felt detoxed and clean after 45 minutes. Wow!

So why is this drug still untested, even though it was approved for clinical trials seventeen years ago? Lack of financial backing has hindered trials, but as drug addiction and alcohol addiction are responsible for such a high percentage of crimes, wouldn't it have been sensible for the US and the UK governments to have financed and instigated these vital trials seventeen years ago? Now in 2007 the FDA are taking this treatment seriously. Yes I am over-simplifying the matter, but I'm sure you'll agree that it's a matter of urgency to find a solution to drug and alcohol addiction! The alkaloid from this plant requires only one shot of the medication to be effective and this treatment can be successful with other addictions including heroin, cocaine, crack cocaine, methadone, alcohol and tobacco. It is available on the internet in capsule form and is legal in the UK, but illegal to possess in the USA, Belgium, Sweden and Switzerland.[77]

If you have a friend or relative who suffers from any of the above addictions you may be able to use your pendulum to help their problem.

Ask your pendulum the following questions:

1. Will a supplement of Ibogaine psychoactive indole alkaloid reduce the craving?
2. You can then ask if the relief is permanent, or if the dose will need to be repeated at intervals?
3. Ibogaine is available from the internet, but you must dowse to check the quality of the capsules.
4. Ask your pendulum if there is any serious health risk from taking this plant?

It is believed that a healthy person will be free of side effects, although it's reported to have a hallucinatory effect for a short time after being taken. This plant is non-addictive and is a treatment free from pharmaceutical chemicals so it's well worth investigating. An addiction can damage both health and family life.

Another plant which has been recognised for centuries as helpful in reducing addiction is Noni. When you have a serious addiction problem it's a case of 'any port in a storm' so when trying to give up an addiction, Noni should be considered. This plant contains a substance called Proxeronine which converts into a critical compound involved in a wide range of normal human biochemical reactions.[79] Dowse and ask if a supplement of Noni will help to reduce symptoms? Also ask if this supplement will benefit health.

This plant has extraordinary healing properties and has been used for over 2,000 years in China, India and Polynesia and other areas to strengthen the immune system and help the body to fight disease. Anyone who has had an addiction for a long period will most likely benefit from this tonic.

References

1. Regenerative Nutrition. Tel. 0845 200 8544.
   http://www.regenerativenutrition.com
2. ibid.
3. Dept. of Neurosurgery, University of Southern California. Keck School of Medicine, Los Angeles, California 90033. Pyrko P., Wang W., Markland F.S., Swenson S.D., Schmitmeier S., Schonthal A.H., Chen TC., http:www.leaddiscovery.co.uk Journal of Neurosurgery. 2005 Sept: 103 (3) 526–37.
4. Nat. Library of Medicine & the National Institute of Health. Anti-tumour activity of cryptophycins: effect of infusion time and combination studies. Menon K., Alvarez E., Forler P., Phares V., Amsrud T., Shih C., Alawar R., Teicher P.A., http://www.ncbi.nlm.gov
5. The Decatur Daily News. Sunday May 1st 2005. 'Scientists Study Scorpion Venum in Cancer Care by Samira Jafari. Associated Press Writer. http://www.decaturdaily.com/decaturdaily/news/050501/scorpion.shtml
6. Marine Biotech.org. Ecteinascidin 734. Cyondelis ® ET-734.
7. Pau D'Arco Tea – There is a Cure for Cancer.
   http://www.pau-d-arco.com
8. The Living Rainforest. 'Cancer Cured by Rosy Periwinkle'.
   http://www.livingrainforest.org
9. BBC News. 30th July 2006. 'Scorpion Venum Attacks Tumours'
10. Nexus Jan. 2007 Vol. 14. No. 1. Letters to the Editor.
11. Nexus New Times Vol. 13. No. 6. Nov. 2006 Sydney Morning Herald. Aug. 28th 2006. http://www.smh.com.au

12. Nexus New Times Vol. 10. No. 5. UK Pure Water Association. http://www.npwa.freeserve.co.uk

13. Nexus New Times May 2007 Vol. 14. No. 3. Source: GM Free Cymuru, http://www.gmfreecymru.org.uk/pivotal_papers/feedingrats.htm. The Independent 11th Feb. 2007 http://tinyurl.com/2dwrff

14. Nexus New Times Vol. 11. No. 5. 'The Hidden Dangers of Soy Allergens' by Kaayla T. Daniel PhD. CCN. From 'The Whole Soy Story', 'The Dark Side of America's Favourite Health Food' New Trends Publishers 2004.

15. Lloyds Pharmacy Ltd. 024 7643 2400 www.lloydspharmacy.com

16. Nexus New Times Vol. 14. No. 1. Tony Hall 'Diabetes 2 is Curable'.

17. Nexus New Times Vol. 11. No. 5. Global News page 7. Independent 27th June 2004. New Scientist Vol. 183 issue 2454 Jkuly 2004.

18. Nexus New Times Vol. 12. No. 4. 'Melanoma of the Skin Not a Sunshine Story' Source: Med Sci Monit, 2004; 10(7) CR336–340 July 1st 2004.

19. MedicineNet.com Alzheimers Disease Overview. Practical information on Alzheimer's. www.medicinenet.com

20. Union of Concerned Scientists. Food, Environment Electronic Digest. April 2006. 'Arsenic in Your Chicken'.

21. Dr Joseph Mercola. The Healing Properties of Raw Honey. www.mercola.com. Yemen News July 7th 2006. BBC News July 7th 2006.

22. *Helping and Healing* by Thomas Haberle. Sheldon Press, London.

23. MedicineNet.com TV Worsens Children's Diabetes. Kids Type1 Diabetes Control Slips with Each Daily TV Hour. By Daniel J. De Noon. WebMD Medical News. Reviewed by Louise Chang MD. http://www.medicinenet.com

24. MicroNutra Health, Scientifically Proven Way to Reduce Your Blood Sugar Level. http://www.micronutra.com

25. MedicineNet.com 'Depression a Treatable Illness' source; National Institute of Health (www.nih.gov)

26. Medical News Today, 'Vaccine Induced Autism Hearings to Present Science Supporting Parents Claim. 5th June 2007. Autism News. The National Autism Association. http://www.nationalautism.org

27. Anticancerinfo.co.uk. Read About the Role of Vitamin B17 in the Fight Against Cancer.

28. Anticancerinfo.co.uk. Patrick Holford. The Institute of Optimum Nutrition. Vitamin B17 in the Fight Against Cancer.

29. MedicineNet. Inc. Ginseng, Flaxseed May Help Cancer Patients. By Amanda Gardner, HealthDay reporter. June 2nd 2007 HealthDay News.

30. Dr Joseph Mercola & Rachael Droege 'How to Avoid the top 10 Most Common Toxins'. www.mercola.com

31. Nexus New Times Vol. 11. No. 6. J.Briggins 'Aspartame Danger'.
32. Electrolytes The Spark of Life by Gillian Martlew MD, study by Elizabeth Reese of the Ministry Laboratory, California. Nature Publishing Ltd.
33. Nexus New Times Vol. 11. No. 4. 'Micro Organisms and Mental Illness' Frank Strick, Clinical Research Director, the Research Inst. For Infectious Mental illness, Santa Cruz.
34. Dr D.Taulbert MD., PhD., University Hospital of Cologne. MedicineNet.com by Miranda Hitti, WebMD. Medical News. Reviewed by Loouise Chang MD., July 3rd 2007. 'Dark Chocolate May Help Blood Pressure' The Journal of the American Medical Association. July 4th 2007. Vol. 298: pp 49–60. News Release JAMA/Archives.
35. Green Health Watch Magazine. www.greenhealthwatch.com 'Alzheimers – New Early Tests' (11869) Heo. H.J., and Lee, C.Y., Journal of Agriculture and Food Chemistry. 2005: 53(5): 1445–48.
36. Green Health Watch Magazine. No. 20. 'Autism Figures Soar in US' The Environmental Health Trust. Forres, Scotland. www.greenhealthwatch.com
37. Holistic News 2133 The Environmental – Health Trust. Green Health Watch. 'Illness of our Time'. http://www.ehn.clara.netwww.greenhealthwatch.com
38. Saxe et al. Journal of American Dental Association, 1999; V130:191. Green Health Watch Magazine. www.greenhealthwatch.com
39. MedicineNet.com HealthDay News. July 5th 2007. 'Key Protein May Explain Men's Higher Liver Cancer Rate'.
40. Sustainable Life. 'EPA's Polyunsaturated Folic Acids – Essential to Health'. http://www.suslife.com
41. ibid.
42. ibid.
43. Dr Joseph Mercola 'Body Absorbs 5lb of Make Up Chemicals Per Year' Telegraph co.uk June 22nd 2007.
44. WEN. The Women's Environmental Network www.wen.org.uk. 'Toxic Tour: What's in my Cosmetics?'
45. Campaign for Safe Cosmetics. 'Safety of Cosmetics is a Gray Area' by Robert Cohen Star-Ledger New Jersey. May 27th 2007.
46. Cystic Fibrosis Foundation 'What You Need to Know About Cystic Fibrosis' http://www.cff.org
47. Courtesy of the Alternative Health Magazine. Winter 2007. http://www.alternativehealth.com 'Holding Alzheimer's in Check'.
48. The Campaign Against Trans Fats in Food www.tfx.org.uk. 'The Dietary Facts and the Risk of Incident Alzheimer's Disease'.
49. Thimerosal & Autism Symptoms Resources, First Official Recognition of Thimerosal Dangers Made May 2003.

www.thimerosal-autism-symptoms.com

50. Womanshealth Channel.com www.tellher.com Sanofi Pasgteur MSD.
51. World
52. World Health Organization. Mental Health. Depression. http://www. WHO.int/mental_health/management/depression/definition/EN.53. Alliance for a Healthy Tomorrow, 'Toxins and our Health', (Excerpted from A Picture of Pollution in People,) written by Michelle Gottlieb and available from Alliance for a Healthy Tomorrow. http://www.healthytomorrow.org
54. Katherine Seligman, chronicle Staff Writer. Feb. 2005. http://www.sfgate.com
55. The World Health Organisation, Skin Cancer How Common is Skin Cancer? Questions and Answers. http://www,who.int/topics/skin_cancer/en/
56. 'You Don't Deserve Brain Cancer –You Deserve The Facts' by Amy Worthington, observer@coldreams.com 26th Feb. 2005. http://www.cam.net.uk
57. The Food Commission March 2007. 'A Spoonful of Sugar'. http://wwwfoodcomm.org.uk/latest_medicines_mar07.htm
58. Campaign for Safe Cosmetics. Feb.2007 'Cancer Causing Chemicals Found in Children's Bath Products'. http://www.safecosmetics.org
59. Campaign for Safe Cosmetics 'Study Finds Industrial Pollution Begins in the Womb, Hundreds of Toxic Chemicals Measured in Newborn Babies' http://www.safecosmetics.org
60. Environmental Defence. 'Asthma Attack'. http://www.environmentaldefence.org
61. Regenerative Nutrition 'Propolis'. http://www.regenerative nutrition.com Dr J.M.N.Grange.
62. ibid.
63. ibid.
64. Asthma UK. For Journalists; 'Key Facts and Statistics'. http://www.asthma.org.uk
65. Courtesy of AlternativeMedicine.com http://www.alternatiemedicine.com 'But Will Medicare Reimburse it?' by James Keough.
66. The Fish Foundation www.fish-foundation.org.uk. 'Omega 3 Fatty Acids in Boys With Behaviour, Learning and Health Problems'.
67. The Nutri Center, 'Eating Disorders – Bulomia Anorexia and Binge-Eating' http://www.avifresh.com Avi Foods System Inc. Source DHHS, NIMH, National Eating Disorders Association.
68. Courtesy of AlternativeMedicine,com 'Heal Thyself – the Inside Scoop-Cranberry Cure – All by James Keough.

69. The New Scientist 7th July 2007. 'Organic Tomatoes Win on Level Farming Field'.
70. Nexus New Times Vol. 14. No. 5. Sept. 2007 'Is the Cause of Cancer a Common Fungus?' by Dr Tullio Simoncini.
71. MedicineNet.com 'Curry Spice may Counter Alzheimers, Chemicals in Curry Sauce may Help Delete Ingredients in Alzheimer's Brain Plaque' by Miranda Hitti, Web MD. Medical News. Reviewed by Brunida Nazario MD. July 16th 2007. http://www.medicinenet.com
72. BBC News, BBC.co.uk. submitted by Babba. Ref. 'Pre-Birth Apples Benefit Babies' Dissect Medicine. http://www.dissectmedicine.com/-story/4468 May 2007.
73. Dr Joseph Mercola. 'Slathering on Sunscreen Does not Prevent Cancer' www.mercola.com
74. Regenerative Nutrition, Wormwood (Artemesia Absinthium). http://www.regenerativenutrion.com
75. The Womens Environmental Network News (WEN) London. www.wen.org.uk
76. The World Health Organisation, Media Centre, 'Diabetes' Fact Sheet F312.
77. Howard S. Lotsof, 'Ibogaine' http://www.ibogaine.co.uk
78. The Campaign for Safe Cosmetics 'Safety of Cosmetics is a Gray Area' by Robert Cohen. Star-Ledger (New Jersey) May 27th 2007-08-08.
79. Regenerative Nutrition. 'Noni Fruit'. http://www.regenerativenutrition.com
80. The National Health Federation 'New Approaches to Alzheimer's Disease and Others' by Dr Russell Blaylock. Autopsy reports on Alzheimer's patients found 70% more aluminium in the brain. http://www.thenhf.com
81. Nexus Jan 2008, Vol. 15 No. 1 Generation Rescue. http://www.generationrescure.org

E-COLI – MRSA – SALMONELLA – FOOD POISONING

Your tummy leaves you in absolutely no doubt when Salmonella is present. The frustrating thing is how easy it is to unwittingly eat contaminated food. When we eat food containing harmful bacteria, quite often it does not affect us immediately – the bacteria has to set up home in your gut, where it produces it's very large family. Bacteria needs moisture and a warm place to grow and as they have a natural ability to divide, in a matter of minutes one becomes two, two become four, and thanks to this exponential growth it doesn't take long before there is a healthy army of millions of bacteria in your gut. This is when you begin to feel the full impact of the invasion. These food bugs have the advantage over us, as we humans cannot see, taste or even smell them. So how can we declare war on this elusive and powerful enemy?

The easiest way is to attack them before they attack you, so my advice is to cleanse the energy of each plate of food, particularly seafood or chicken, before you eat it. This is done by simply holding your hands over the plate of food for a second while you mentally visualise a beam of white light passing through the food, and mentally ask for it to be cleansed of the vibration of all chemicals and harmful bacteria.

This may sound complicated but once you have done the exercise a few times, you will find that it only takes a second or two for the thought to flash through your mind! This exercise is useful to boost the energy of food which has been in transit for days and perhaps grown in soil treated with powerful chemicals. If you do not believe that my advice is correct, dowse for confirmation!

Attack is the best method of defence as once these bacteria have incubated (which can be anything from a few hours to a few days), you develop powerful symptoms which can include violent sickness, diarrhoea and very nasty tummy pains. How do you diagnose when you have food poisoning and when you have MRSA?[13] How do you diagnose which bug has attacked you?

Dowse and ask if your symptoms are caused by harmful bacteria in your gut? Then ask your pendulum if the culprit is E Coli? Salmonella? Campylobacter? Clostridium Perfrigens? Listeria or MRSA? Ask each question separately and you will be able to diagnose the cause of your discomfort.

Colloildal Silver is an excellent treatment to kill almost all harmful bacteria in the gut and can be purchased from health stores. This tasteless liquid is also an effective treatment for skin infections, so a useful addition to your medicine cabinet. Another powerful bacteria killer is Grapefruit Seed Extract which can kill all known bacteria. This natural extract kills all tummy bugs but it also kills good bacteria, so if you're taking this cure, it is important to replace friendly bacteria in your gut by eating natural yoghurt.

Dowse and ask the following questions:

1. Will a course of Colloidal Silver kill the harmful bacteria in my gut?
2. Will a course of Grapefruit Seed Extract kill the harmful bacteria in my gut.

You can then dowse and ask which is the more beneficial of the two treatments.

As well as E Coli, there are other food borne illnesses which can disrupt your social life. We regularly read articles reminding us that certain fish may contain mercury, but perhaps the poor fish have another serious problem!

In China, many fish are raised in sewage infested waters and to make matters worse, in order to compensate for the lack of clean water, antibiotics, pesticides and fungicides are pumped into the water.

Many of these fish are imported to the USA and this year the US has increased their import of these fish by 34%. If you regularly eat fish for dinner then dowsing is a 'must' to establish if the fish has any harmful contents.

1. Ask the question 'Does this fish contain mercury?' If 'Yes' you can ask the pendulum to please remove the mercury and show you the 'Yes' sign when finished.
2. 'Does this fish contain harmful bacteria?'
3. 'Does the fish contain (a) pesticides, (b) fungicides or (c) antibiotics?' If you receive a 'Yes' answer, you have the option of dowsing to establish if it is a, b or c, or placing the fish in the garbage bin. Please do not feed it to your cat!

Are these unfortunate fish from China part of the reason that one in every four Americans suffer a food borne illness and roughly 20% of cases are due to contaminated seafood?[3]

Dowse and ask your pendulum if some of the seafood imported from China is responsible for certain food borne illnesses? Seafood often contains mercury and can 'go off' when left in a warm kitchen, so it is important to dowse your seafood before eating it to avoid an unpleasant tummy upset.

Salmonella is caused by the presence of the salmonella bacteria in certain foods, the most likely being seafood, poultry, eggs, meat or raw milk.

Foodborn illnesses are rising in number each year in the West and in the USA roughly 76 million cases of this illness occur each year. The World Health Organization reports that of this number, 325,999 are hospitalised and 5,000 die.[10] To say Salmonella is thriving is an understatement. It's hard to believe but there are over 2,500 known types of the salmonella bacteria and overuse of antibiotics has created a bacteria which is multi-drug resistant.[12]

Are you suffering from sickness, diarrhoea and nasty tummy pains? Then it's time to dowse to ask:

1. Are you suffering from Salmonella? If you receive a 'No' then ask your pendulum the next question.
2. Are your symptoms caused by a foodborn illness? If you receive a 'Yes' answer, ask the next question.
3. Are my symptoms caused by Campylobacter bacteria?

Campylobacter

Campylobacter is a nasty bacteria which can cause serious diarrhoea illness and is a well known cause of gastro enteritis. This unfriendly bacteria certainly makes its presence known as the sufferer can experience fever, nausea, vomiting and severe tummy pains.

Dowsing will enable you to diagnose whether your symptoms are caused by a foodborne or airborne bacteria, and confirm the best treatment to relieve and reduce the symptoms.

Arsenicam relieves symptoms of sea food poisoning. Other effective treatments are Echinacea, garlic and tea tree oil. Myrrh is an antibiotic along with horseradish, watercress and nasturtiums. Colloidal silver is also very effective as it kills most bacteria. For difficult to remove bacteria, you can drink a few drops of grapefruit seed extract as this kills all known bacteria. The only problem, as I mentioned earlier, is that as it kills all bacteria it also kills the good bacteria in your body, so it is important to replace it. This can be done by eating natural yoghurt.

Dowse and ask which of the above treatments is right for your body.

MRSA – Methicillin Resistant Stephylococcus Aureus

The MRSA bug seems to be thriving in many hospitals in the UK and claiming the lives of patients while making others very ill. This bug seems to always be one jump ahead of the medical profession as it has developed an immunity to powerful antibiotics.

Those who've had surgery are most at risk as it specialises in infecting surgical wounds. Perhaps a natural treatment is the last weapon against this powerful bug.

Dr Ron Cutler, a microbiologist from the University of East London, has shown in research that this bug can be killed within days with the use of Allicin which occurs naturally in garlic. This research was carried out in 2003, which makes you wonder why MRSA is still thriving in hospitals.[17]

Last week I visited my local hospital and was amazed to see large notices displayed stating only next of kin were allowed to visit in wards due to this virus. We are now in 2008. Perhaps it's time for hospitals to try alternative treatments in this war against MRSA.

If you know anyone who is unfortunate enough to suffer from this illness then dowse and ask the following questions:

1. Can Allicin in garlic kill the MRSA?
2. Will balancing the negative and positive ions in the building kill the virus? Research on industrial ionisers showed that the MRSA virus could not survive in atmosphere which had a high level of negative ions.
3. Does this virus thrive in the presence of positive ions?

When you have suffered severe sickness, your body is likely to be short of minerals and vitamins. Dowse and ask if your body would benefit from a combined supplement of minerals and vitamins? Also ask if your body's acid/alkaline level is out of balance, as violent vomiting over a few days can disturb tummy acids.

Manuka honey has been recognised for its healing qualities for many centuries and today hospitals in many parts of the world use it to treat wounds. The great benefit of using honey to treat injuries and infection is that this natural antibiotic is free from side effects.

The Washington Post reports that MRSA has met its match. According to the Center of Disease Control and Prevention, Manuka honey has shown great promise when treating wounds infected with superbug MRSA, whose incidence has increased 32 fold in US hospitals in recent years.

The European Journal of Medical Research reported in 2003 that honey had an 85% success rate in treating infected post-Caesarean wounds compared with 50% success rate of conventional intervention.[14]

If a member of your family is suffering from MRSA in a wound, dowse and ask:

1. Will Manuka honey placed on the wound remove the superbug?
2. Will Manuka honey kill harmful bacteria in a wound?

It's always nice to hear that grandma's home remedies are still reliable and now being accepted by the medical profession to replace antibiotics, which seem powerless in their fight against super microbes.

Research has shown that the MRSA virus thrives in areas where the level of positive ions are present and of course hospitals have lots of electrical equipment and therefore have a high level of positive ions. Using an industrial ioniser will reduce the level of these ions and help to introduce more negative ions into the building.

Dowse and ask if the MRSA virus thrives in areas where there is a high level of positive ions? If you receive a 'Yes' answer, then dowse and ask if installing the right number of industrial ionisers will reduce the number of instances of MRSA virus in hospitals?

EAR PROBLEMS

Ears – Ringing

Ringing in the ears can be linked to a manganese deficiency, so ask your pendulum if the ringing in your ears would be reduced by including manganese in your diet.

Ears – Middle ear problem

Check if your body is short of manganese. If you receive a 'Yes' then ask the pendulum if the middle ear problems will be reduced when you include manganese in your diet.

ELEPHANTITUS

Fortunately this illness is not very common in the West but it causes a lot of heartache to sufferers. What is the cause of this unusual illness?

I am told that the culprit is the presence of the worm Filaria, so dowse and ask if this worm is the cause of this illness? Dowse and ask if Gingko biloba will be helpful? Dowse and would Grapefruit Seed Extract kill this parasite?

The World Health Organization report that over 120,000 million sufferers of this disfiguring illness are confirmed to be caused by a thread-like parasite: the Filarial worm. These worms live in the lymphatic system of infected humans and the illness is spread by mosquitoes that bite the infected person and then pass on the infection.[11]

Yesterdays TV news reported this year 2007 would see an increase in mosquitoes in UK due to the excessive rain, so let's hope only the uninfected ones breed here!

ENDOMETRIOSIS

Many experts believe that most cases of Endometriosis are linked to environmental toxins, dioxins and other pollutants. Are they to blame? Today, many illnesses are blamed on dioxins and certain environmental toxins. These illnesses include Asthma, Chronic Fatigue Syndrome, Diabetes and some cancers.

It's recognised that if a person is sleeping over Geopathic Stress then their immune system is being weakened which will destroy their body's resistance to illness and make them more susceptible to these negative toxins.

Dioxins are a large group of over 70 chemicals found in our environment which come from industrial processes including smelting, incineration and bleaching of paper. We are all vulnerable to these chemicals as they are in the atmosphere and can affect anyone whose immune system is low. As well as being in the atmosphere and being a threat to humans, they are also a threat to animals, which in turn increases their affect on us – they land on animals which form an important part of our food chain.

Dowse and ask your pendulum if your Endometriosis is linked to environmental toxins? Then ask if you were sleeping over Geopathic Stress prior to when you developed the illness?

Another group of toxins which are associated with illnesses are PCB's which come from insulation, coolants and non-inflammable chemicals. Dowse and ask if PCB's are a cause of your illness?

Many doctors blame the presence of the Flatworm as a cause of this illness, so dowse and ask if the Flat Worm is present in your body? If you receive a 'Yes' answer, you can purchase a product from the health shop to remove them from your system.

Another enemy is carbohydrates as excessive carbohydrates in the diet can kill Amylase, the friendly enzyme. Ask the pendulum if your body is short of this enzyme?

Dowse and ask if any of the following supplements will improve the symptoms? (1) Selenium, (2) Wild Yam, (3) Agnus Castus, (4) Zinc, (5) Essential Fatty Acids, (6) Calcium, (7) Magnesium or (8) Vitamins B, C or E.

EPILEPSY

Epilepsy affects people in many parts of the world. This neurological disorder causes the sufferer to experience uncontrollable muscle jerking.

In some parts of the world, unfortunate sufferers are thought to be attacked by an unseen force but this is not the cause of the spasms. Doctors now know that Epileptic fits are linked to action of brain cells; a breakdown in the electrical activity of the brain causes motor sensory problems.

The World Health Organization reports between 50,000 and 100,000 incidences of epilepsy each year and, interestingly, they report different causes of the problem. In Latin America, the common cause is Neurocysticercosis cysts on the brain which come from tapeworm infection.

In Africa, malaria and meningitis are blamed while in India, Tuberculosis is often linked to this illness.[9] What is the cause of Epilepsy in the West?

Dowse and ask your pendulum the following.

1. Is the epilepsy linked to the presence of a worm?
2. Is it linked to damage done by sleeping over Geopathic Stress?
3. Does the sufferer have an Acid/Alkaline pH imbalance?
4. Ask if a supplement of potassium will reduce seizures.
5. Does the body have an excess of Copper? If you receive a 'Yes' then sit down and ask the pendulum to please remove this excess and balance the level. Also ask if the Zinc level is balanced, as Copper and Zinc interact.

Gran Mal Fit can be caused by a Magnesium or Calcium deficiency. Also, check if patient's body is short of Manganese? Ask your pendulum is they are short of the amino acid Taurine? And are they short of Vitamin B6? Would the plant Sculcap be of benefit?

Dowse and ask if the sufferer is sleeping over Geopathic Stress?

EYE PROBLEMS

Eyes – Night blindness

Night vision can be improved by including blueberries or red grapes in your diet as they contain anthocyanins. Bilberry supplement and blackcurrant jam also work to improve night vision. This improvement has been reported within 30 minutes of taking the berries. Night blindness can sometimes be linked to a deficiency of Zinc, so dowse and check if your body is short.

Eyes – Cataracts

Cataracts are a common eye problem suffered mainly by the elderly. Many describe it as the lens of the eyes becoming cloudy. It's a bit like looking through a steamed up window in the kitchen after cooking the dinner or the magical frost pattern on a winter's morning. The symptoms are caused by a calcium deposit collecting on the optic nerve.

Removal of a cataract today is a safe and effective surgical procedure that can be carried out when the cataract seriously affects your vision.

Many folks blame this condition on damage caused by free radicals, while others place the blame on too many dairy foods in the diet. Dowse and ask if your cataract is caused by free radicals in the environment? If you receive a 'No' answer then ask if the cataract is caused by excess dairy foods in your diet?

The herb Eyebright to the rescue! This herb is well known as a safe treatment for cataracts and can be taken orally or as an eye drop.

First, dowse and ask if any of the following will reduce the cataract. If you receive a 'Yes' answer, ask about each of them separately. (1) Bilberry, (2) Vitamin A, (3) Vitamin B12, (4) Vitamin E, (5) Zinc, (6) Rutin, (7) Elderflower, (8) Thyme, (9) Selenium, (10) L. Glutamine, (11) Amino Acids Lysine, Glutathione or Lutien.

MSM Organic Sulphur is a versatile treatment that can be used to improve arthritis symptoms, emphysema distress and airborne allergens like Hay Fever, but MSM can also be used to treat Cataracts.[1]

Regenerative Nutrition reports that bathing the eye in a solution of 15% MSM has been found to reverse cataracts. Dowse and ask your pendulum if your cataract will be reduced by regularly bathing the eye in MSM Organic Sulphur solution? Including vitamin C in your diet can often help prevent a cataract.

If you have a cataract problem, before going through the ordeal of having an eye operation, consider altering your diet to include more alkaline and less acid food.

Acid in the body is linked to the calcium deposits, so by balancing the acid/alkaline level, it helps your body to release excess deposits.

Dowse and ask the following questions:

1. Is there an acid/alkaline imbalance in your body?
2. Is an excess of acid linked to the cataract problem?
3. Is the acid/alkaline imbalance linked to the macular degeneration?

You can ask the pendulum to correct the acid/alkaline pH balance, but it will only be temporary. To improve the balance you must include more fruit and green vegetables in your diet and replace coffee with herbal tea, as this will quickly help to balance the acid level in your body.

The enzyme Serrapeptase could very well be the answer to many eye problems. This amazing enzyme from the silk worm has the ability to reduce inflammation and remove scar tissue and blood clots. It has a great track record when taken as a pill or capsule on an empty stomach. Dowse and ask if Serrapeptase can improve your eyesight problem.

Eyes – Detached retina

A detached retina is a serious problem and Lutein may be of assistance. This cartenoid protects the macula (central retina) from blue and ultraviolet light.

A detached retina in dogs has been found to be linked to a deficiency of Zinc and Taurine and while you are a human and not a dog, it may be worth exploring this possibility. Ask your pendulum if your body is short of zinc? Also ask if a supplement of amino acid Taurine will improve this eye problem?

Dry eyes

Omega 3 fish oil found in sardines, cod and mackerel is a great source of DHA (docosahexaenioc acid), which supports cell membranes and helps with dry eyes and macular degeneration.

Silica and phytoestrol (rhubarb extract) are both reported to benefit dry eyes along with the amino acid Taurine.

Eyes – Glaucoma

Glaucoma is a nasty eye problem. It creeps up silently and is often established before it is diagnosed. It creates serious pressure inside the eye, which can damage the optic nerve.

Eyebright drops, derived from the plant Eyebright, are an excellent natural treatment.

Vitimin A is also helpful, as well as Bilberry which protects blood vessels and delicate veins in the eyes. It can be taken in tablet form.

Ginkgo Biloba is an excellent remedy as it helps the oxygen supply to reach the eyes and therefore increase the circulation there. An added bonus is that this ancient tree has the ability to reduce harmful toxins.

Zinc sulphate has healing qualities and can delay vision loss.

Beta Carotene, Selenium, vitamins A, B12, C and E, Bilberry, and the amino acid Taurine all halt deterioration. Dowse each one separately.

Many cataract sufferers claim that smoking cannabis lowers the ocular pressure, so dowse and ask if this plant has the ability to reduce the ocular pressure in your eye?

Dowse and ask if alcohol aggravates this eye problem?

Eyes – Macular degeneration

Macular degeneration is one of the problems associated with old age! One cause can be scar tissue from a cataract, which can possibly be removed by taking a course of Serrapeptose. This amazing natural treatment has the ability to eat dead tissue in the body and so give relief.

The amino acid Taurine, as well as helping glaucoma suffers, is known to help halt molecular degeneration. Bilberry extract, selenium, beta carotene and vitamins A, B12, C and E are all beneficial. Gingko biloba can increase the circulation to the back of the eyes and is therefore a useful addition to eye care. Dowse each of the above to ask which would be beneficial to reduce your cataract.

Dowse and ask if taking a dose of magnesium at bedtime each evening will help to maintain blood to the eyes and brain, thereby halting macular degeneration?

Eggs are a rich source of sulphur, so including them in your diet will help to protect the eye lenses from cataract formation as they contain lecithin, cysteine and lutien. Dowse and ask if eggs in your diet will help to improve your eye health.

Eyes twitching

Twitching eyes can be due to a lack of calcium. If you are troubled by an annoying twitching of your eye lid, then dowse and ask the pendulum if your body is short of calcium?

Eyes – Conjunctivitis

This eye problem is usually cleared up quickly as it responds to both natural and medical treatment. Symptoms of this eye problem include red eyes and irritation which is caused by an inflammation of the membrane. Some sufferers complain of a burning sensation and a sticky discharge is often present.

Dowse and ask the pendulum if Calendula can reduce symptoms? Calendula, which is a natural antiseptic, is a soothing treatment that will reduce the upsetting itchiness while also reducing inflammation. It is available from most health shops.

Chamomile has healing properties and Vitamin A and is important for healthy eyes.

An old wives' cure is to place a slice of raw potato on each eye in order to relieve the symptoms. This is not as daft as it sounds – a slice of raw potato placed on a skin blemish is known to help heal, and what about a slice of cucumber to refresh the eyes? Many women use this old trick to rejuvenate tired eyes before an evening out.

Dowse and ask if Fennel, Chamomile or Colloidal silver could be beneficial? Also dowse and ask if bathing your eyes in a solution of Colloidal Silver will help to kill the infection?

FIBROMYALGIA (FMA)

Fibromyalgia is a modern day illness which is affecting an ever increasing number of sufferers in the western world. There doesn't seem to be one specific cause of this debilitating illness as it can be blamed on trauma or the modern day diet of food containing toxins and harmful chemicals.

I question the suggestion that such a high number of sufferers could develop the illness based on experienced trauma. Previous generations lived through much greater trauma, the 40's war and the London Blitz, so why did symptoms not appear then? Folks did however have a healthier diet, free from chemicals, suggesting perhaps modern day chemicals are linked to this illness.

Dowse and ask:

1. Is Fibromyalgia caused by experiencing trauma?
2. Is it caused by a diet containing toxins and harmful chemicals?
3. Is Fibromyalgia caused by electromagnetic energy?

Some doctors believe that excessive carbohydrates in the diet cause a depletion of the enzyme Amylase. As this enzyme helps the carbohydrate to digest in the body, problems could occur.

Dowse and ask if some of the pain can be linked to undigested waste from carbohydrate consumption?

Any Fibromyalgia sufferer will tell you that this modern day illness is the scourge of the century. Within the past fifteen years this complaint has made its presence felt in the Western world. In the USA alone there are several million sufferers. Symptoms can vary from person to person and can include stiffness and chronic ache, tender spots, muscular-skeletal pains and unexplained fatigue.

Very often sufferers will experience menstrual pains and cramps and complain that ligaments, tendons and muscles will be very painful for no apparent reason.

Sleep is often disturbed by aches when lying in one position for a time or by sudden violent cramp or twitching legs, so getting a good night's sleep is a real problem. Sleep is critical to good health so a supplement is essential and this is where dowsing is helpful – it eliminates the trial and error syndrome.

A low level of Melatonin is helpful to improve sleep but do not take a high level, no matter how desperately tired you may feel, as this could cause you to feel drowsy into the following day. Melatonin is not on sale in the UK but is available in the USA and on the internet.

Due to the pain and lack of energy, it is very difficult to attend any form of alternative group which may help to relieve pain. However, sufferers have found that Pilates helps relieve the pain and improve health, and Yoga reduces the level of stress in the body.

Dowse and ask the following questions:

1. Would a supplement of Melatonin improve my sleep pattern?
2. Would a supplement of Brewers Yeast improve my health?
3. Will regular Pilates exercise improve FMA symptoms?
4. Can Yoga exercise reduce the level of stress in my body?
5. Would Amylase (a friendly enzyme) relieve symptoms?
6. Does excess carbohydrate in the diet aggravate the symptoms?
7. Would a supplement of the amino acid S-Adenosyl-methione (SAM) benefit my health?
8. Would a supplement of Germanium improve the symptoms?
9. Dowse and ask if the person is sleeping over Geopathic Stress.

Some sufferers firmly believe that Fibromyalgia is caused by the presence of Mercury in their body introduced by a vaccination. This is an interesting thought as it would certainly account for the high number of folks stricken with this illness. Dowse and ask if Fibromyalgia is linked to Mercury in a vaccination? You can then rephrase the question and ask if Mercury in a vaccination is a cause of Fibromyalgia symptoms?

FLATULENCE

The Scottish poet Robert Burn wrote 'Let Air Gang Free Where ere You Be' but alas any sufferer will tell you that this advice is not always convenient! A regular problem of flatulence can often be linked to the presence of bacterial overgrowth in the gastrointest-inal tract.

These parasites can cause inadequate digestive juices to be secreted by the stomach, pancreas or gall bladder. Dowse and ask if parasites reside in your body? You'll find lots of medications on sale in a pharmacy, so dowse to ask which medication is the most suitable for your body and which one will resolve the prob-lem. You can also dowse to ask if the body is short of Amylase, a friendly enzyme, and if Parsley Tea will treat the symptoms.

Dowse and ask if taking a supplement of Colloidal Silver for a few days will remove the parasites? Now dowse and ask if taking a course of Grape Fruit Seed Extract will remove the parasites?

FREE RADICALS AND ANTIOXIDANTS

What are Free Radicals? They are the 'Bad Guys'. Always be on your guard against Free Radicals as they declare war on the good cells in our blood and speed up the ageing process! We all get old soon enough and we don't want assistance from Free Radicals! They come from toxic substances including pesticides in food, pollution and mental or physical stress.

Fortunately Mother Nature gave us Antioxidants which play a vital part in protecting the cells in our body from these Free Radi-cals. Selenium is an excellent antioxidant and a valuable part of our diet.

GALLSTONES

Many therapists today are advising against having keyhole surgery as it is reported on certain occasions to cause gall to leak to surrounding tissue.

Magnesium is recognised for its properties of stopping stones from forming. Dowse and ask if your body is short of Magnesium?

Cranberry has a great record for dissolving stones. Lecithin is also known to dissolve stones, while balancing cholesterol and is needed by the gallbladder. Bearberry also has the ability to dissolve stones and apple juice can soften them. Carrot and beetroot are also helpful for this painful problem.

Devil's Claw Root Tea is a favourite with many sufferers along with Holly tea, which dissolves small stones. The amino acid Taurine is also helpful to release stones and the advice from many doctors is to drink plenty of water.

Dowse and ask which of the following will most quickly dissolve your gallstones? (1) Cranberry Juice, (2) Bearberry, (3) Apple Juice, (4) Carrot, (5) Beetroot, (6) Lecithin, (7) Taurine, (8) Devil's Claw Root Tea, (9) Holly Tea.

A friend who suffered from Gall bladder problems told me his secret to deal with the problem was to sleep on the left side rather than the right side as this allowed grit to move in the bladder. He explained it was all about the laws of gravity!

WHAT'S HAPPENING TO THE HUMAN GENES?

The subject of the human genome looks set for an 'all change' view. Until now, scientists have believed that human genes all operate independently of each other and that certain genes were linked to certain illnesses and strengths.

Well here's something interesting to dowse. Revelations in the human genome field suggest that perhaps scientists have had it all wrong since 1973 when DNA was first discovered.

New findings suggest that genes operate in a complex network and interact with each other. If science has got it wrong and each gene is not linked to a specific illness, it's back to the drawing board!

This new information creates an interesting slant on GE crops; in many of these food crops, one gene has been added for a specific function, so this is food for thought! The most interesting fact about this change in genome thinking is that patents will also need rethinking – if genes don't work separately, the details on the patients will be wrong! A very interesting dowsing exercise!

If genes do not work separately, then what effect will it have on our health to be regularly eating processed food which has a foreign gene? The side effects are unknown and as it is early days for symptoms to be linked to genes, it may be a few years before the presence of symptoms and the presence of foreign genes is recognised.

Dr Joseph Mercola reports that roughly 75% of processed food on sale in the USA contains genetically altered ingredients.[15] This new thinking could well be opening an enormous can of worms. Will we begin to see lots of legal cases on the flawed gene theory?

Dowse and ask the following questions:

1. Has science misunderstood the interaction of human genes?
2. Where a foreign gene has been inserted into food, could it ever create illness?
3. Will genes inserted into food be able to interact with genes not present in the food?
4. Is it possible to remove foreign genes from the body?

Many foods have been genetically altered to include unlikely genes. For example, rice containing human genes is now being grown. What effect will this have on health? More worryingly, will there be an antidote for any illness created by the presence of foreign genes in our body?

This is an alarming subject and I am certain you will be able to think of a great many questions to dowse regarding the long term effect of gene manipulation.

Will we soon be eating our genes?

I could fill an entire book on the subject of genetic engineering and genes being used to alter animals and plants, but I will give you only one example.

Can rice containing human genes be good for our health? Does it mean we could be eating a non-compatible gene? There are lots of questions people are asking about these and similar crops. In Missouri, 270 acres of rice were grown. Although this rice looked very normal, it was anything but – it was engineered to produce two pharmaceutical compounds Lactoferrin and Lyso-zyme, both of which are derived from human genes.[18]

Had any of those involved in the birth of this crop stopped to consider if any of 'we humans' may have a violent reaction to this rice? If this happened, do they have an antidote? As with all genetically altered crops, there is a constant danger of cross polli-nation with normal crops, which is a hidden health hazard. We could see health problems ahead. Doctors are not equipped to diagnose illnesses caused by these unknown gene cocktails and this subject is not yet included in the medical school curriculum!

Dowse and ask the following questions:

1. Can rice containing these pharmaceutical compounds from human genes cause an allergic reaction?
2. Is there any benefit to human health from consuming this rice which contains pharmaceutical compounds from human genes?
3. Is it possible for the pharmaceutical compound containing human genes to interact with genes not in the rice crop?
4. Could it cause unknown illnesses for which there is no known cure?

Remember, we have been informed of the discovery by scien-tists that all genes interact with each other, so should scientists really be placing unnatural genes in food crops? And is there any way these compounds could affect our DNA?

Your DNA

We have all heard of DNA and know that this new science can be used to identify criminals, but what exactly is DNA? The name DNA is an abbreviation of Deoxyribonucleic Acid – the basic building block of all human beings. Human DNA is a coding system of our genes and an instruction manual for the four different kinds of nucleotides; the code of life. DNA personalises each one of us, as every human being has their own special indi-vidual combination and sequence of nucleotides and cells. The DNA contains four different letters and this combination of

letters shows that each cell in the body contains a subtle difference. This combination of letters is drawn from a three billion
letter manual. And I thought 'Scrabble' was difficult!

Today DNA can be altered by scientists moving genes around
in animals and plants, but can they alter human genes?

Ask your pendulum the questions:

1. Are there any chemicals in the environment which can alter
   human genes?
2. Is it possible for the DNA to be altered without our knowledge?

Genes

What is happening to our genes? Who can explain why there
are considerably fewer boys than girls being born in some
countries, including America and Japan? Is the culprit the
'gender bender' chemical Nonyphenol Ethoxylates (NPE's)?
NPE's are recognised as potent endocrine disrupters and are
thought to be responsible for male fish transforming into
female in many waterways around the world.

Dr Mercola reports that NPE's can affect genes by turning
them Off and On, thus interfering with the body's glandular
system. This makes me want to ask the question 'Why are
approximately 400 million pounds of this lethal chemical being
manufactured each year?'[16]

Dowse and ask the following questions:

1. Can NPE's disrupt the endocrine glands?
2. Do NPE's affect gene expression?
3. Do they mimic the female hormone estrogen?
4. Do these toxins build up in your system?

These chemical toxins are found in many household detergents
and cleaning agents, so dowse to find which products contain
these harmful chemicals. Whoever said the words 'Good clean
dirt doesn't do you any harm' was perhaps talking more sense
than they realised!

GEOPATHIC STRESS (GS)

Geopathic Stress (GS) is an invisible energy which rises from underground streams and rock cracks several hundred feet underground. When this energy is present in your home or workplace, it can weaken your immune system. This silent energy rises either in a line or a spiral and if your bed happens to be situated on this energy line, the constant bombardment of this negative energy for eight hours each night will weaken your immune system. As a result, your body has less resistance to illness and viruses.

You often hear people saying 'Ever since I moved to this house, I seem to have one illness after another,' or 'I always seem to be tired since I moved to this house'. These are sure signs that you are sleeping or sitting over Geopathic Stress energy for as well as attacking you while you sleep, this energy can attack you when you sit for several hours each day at a desk or on a settee watching television.

The interesting thing about this energy is that the lines can travel down one side of the bed and not the other side, so the wife can constantly complain of feeling tired or suffer from all sorts of unexplained aches and pains, while the husband remains unaffected by the energy. It is possible to have several GS lines running under your home, all moving in different directions and at different depths below your home. Serious health trouble arises when two of these negative lines cross. This creates a double strength negative energy, which is linked to many health problems.

I have been clearing homes of Geopathic Stress for nearly twenty years and in that time I have found that every patient who suffered from cancer, heart disease or other major illnesses slept over the point where these lines crossed. These findings have been confirmed by several experts in various parts of the world.

Kathe Bachler in her book '*Earth Radiation*' describes how the homes of 3,000 children who all suffered from learning difficulties were tested and in 98% of cases they were found to be sleeping over Geopathic Stess energy.[20] Rolf Gordon in his reports in his excellent book *Are You Sleeping in a Safe Place* that confirmation comes from Dr F.S. Andersen. His Cancer Clinic arranged for the homes of 300 cancer patients to be checked for GE, and again the energy was found in these homes.

Dr Hans Nieper reports that 92% of all the cancer patients he treated over several years all slept over Geopathic Stress.[19]

Perhaps the most famous expert on this powerful energy was Gustav Freiherr von Pohl who wrote *Earth Currents, Causative Factor of Cancer and Other Diseases* in 1983. In 1929 he dowsed and located homes where cancer sufferers had lived, and made a valiant effort to get the health effects of Geopathic Stress recognised.

It's been a slow road but nowadays, builders in parts of Austria and Germany must dowse a building for this energy before planning permission is given, and in some areas of Germany the builder must guarantee that sleeping and living accommodation is free from Geopathic Stress.

This energy has been linked to Cancer for many decades and although the energy itself does not give you an illness, it does play havoc with your immune system so that your body is rendered unable to fight illness.

Young children are very sensitive to energy and many mothers are puzzled why their young baby snuggles up cramped in one corner of the cot and each time they place them in the centre of the cot, they work their way back into a corner. These babies sense the negative energy and move as far away from it as possible. The same situation applies with young children who do not want to sleep on their bed and keep climbing out of bed to sleep on the floor. It is not that they are being naughty, it's simply because they recognise the energy is not healthy. Yes, there are a few children who play up and decide it is fun to sleep on the floor but it's important to dowse if your child has a preference for the floor. Try moving the cot or bed and see if the problem stops.

Certain animals are also affected by this energy, while others seem to thrive on it. Dogs will often refuse to sleep on their bed if it is over a bad energy line and horses will not settle if their stable is over a line. Sheep and cows will avoid this energy and if cows are housed in a barn which is over the energy, their milk supply will be depleted and their health will deteriorate. Although most animals in our life avoid this energy, cats are the exception. For some reason they are drawn to this energy and even though it is bad for their health they will make every effort to sit on an energy line. Some vets believe the increase in Leukaemia in cats is due to them sleeping over these lines.

It is time to dowse and ask if Geopathic Stress energy is in your home.

1. Are any Geopathic Stress energy lines running across my home? If you receive a 'Yes' answer then ask the following questions.
2. Am I sleeping over a GS energy line?
3. Is any member of my immediate family sleeping over GS energy?
4. Now ask if you are working over a GS energy line.
5. Ask if any member of your immediate family is working over a GS line.
6. Are any of my animals sleeping over a GS line?

It is possible to clear this energy from your home with the aid of a pendulum. Start by cleansing your energy field by bringing white light down around you to wash away any negative energy which may be clinging to your aura.

It is so easy for negative energy to attach to you when you are standing in a supermarket next to a person who has had a violent row with their boss or has financial worries, so always cleanse your energy field before using the pendulum to cleanse energy or channel medication. You are probably convinced your energy field does not need cleansing, but a cleanse is always beneficial. Once you have cleansed your energy field, it is time to cleanse the energy of the pendulum to ensure it works efficiently.

Simply visualise a bean of white light passing through the pendulum or send it a blast of healing or Reiki energy to cleanse it.

Now it is time to ask your pendulum to please clear your home of Geopathic Stress and to show you the 'Yes' sign when the work has been done. This may take five minutes so be patient. You'll be glad you made the effort to say good bye to this negative energy.

Are you wondering why so many more buildings are now being affected by this energy than ever before? I am told on good authority that the reason there is so much more Geopathic Stress in homes is that in the 1950's, when all the atomic bomb testing was taking place, the enormous force of these bombs damaged the Earth's protective shell. As a result, today there are many small cracks which allow the negative energy to rise into our homes. This explanation certainly makes a lot of sense, so dowse and ask your pendulum if the atomic bomb explosions damaged the Earth's protective layer.

If you would like to learn more about this fascinating subject I recommend Rolf Gordon's book *Are You Sleeping in a Safe Place* as it has been well researched and is written in easy to understand language.

GUILLIAN-BARR SYNDROME

Guillian-Barr Syndrome is a painful autoimmune system illness which upsets the body's defences and causes the immune system to declare war on the nervous system. This creates damaged and severely inflamed nerves and causes weakness in the muscles.

Many sufferers are sleeping over Geopathic Stress energy and have a weak immune system, but what else causes the sufferer to develop this illness?

It is often blamed on the Measles Virus, so dowse and ask if the Measles virus is linked to this syndrome? Also ask the pendulum if the sufferer would benefit from a supplement of Pfaffia.

Ask your pendulum if it is possible to remove the vibration of the measles virus by dowsing. If you receive a 'Yes' answer, cleanse the pendulum and ask it to please remove the vibration of the measles virus from the person, and show you the 'Yes' sign when finished.

GOITER

A goiter is very often linked to the thyroid gland and symptoms appear when this gland is enlarged. Many goiters are linked to an iodine deficiency, so dowse and ask if your body is short of iodine.

A simple test I use to check if my body is short of iodine is to purchase a small bottle of iodine tincture from the pharmacist and paint a small amount roughly the size of a pea, on the inside of my wrists each night. Some people paint the tincture on the inside of their thigh where it is less conspicuous. If the body is short of iodine it will be absorbed within 12 hours and if the yellow stain remains on the skin after this time, your body is not absorbing extra iodine. It is telling you it has a sufficient level.

It may sound strange to paint the tincture on your skin but remember the skin is the largest organ in the body and it absorbs a high percent of most of the ingredients placed on the skin which then go into the bloodstream.

GOUT

Gout can be caused by excess uric acid which causes a blockage. It can also be caused by an infection of the lymphatic vessel due to rich living.

Fresh Tomatoes are known to enable the patient to pass uric acid through the body, and Celery seeds are also able to instigate the passing of uric acid through the body. Devil's Claw Root Tea purifies the blood and Flax Seed Oil can increase the flow of oxygen.

Dowse and ask if eating fresh tomatoes will clear the uric acid blockage and if you receive a 'No' answer then ask if eating Celery Seeds will clear the gout.

You can also dowse and ask your pendulum if Lethicin, Pfaffia, Nettles or Goutwort will relieve the symptoms. Pfaffia is a great supplement for many health problems so will almost certainly help relieve Gout.

Some doctors advise sufferers to avoid drinking port or eating asparagus, so you can dowse and ask if drinking a glass of port will instigate an attack of gout? And then ask if eating asparagus can instigate an attack of gout?

We all know that rich food is often blamed as the cause of gout, but eating red meat, poultry, rich puddings and good booze are only a factor if the diet does not include fresh fruit and green vegetables to balance the pH level. When an attack of gout erupts it is often caused by having eaten the wrong food, as it erupts when the body's Acid/Alkaline level is out of balance.

Dowse and ask the following questions:

1. Is the acid/alkaline level in my body balanced?
2. Is the acid level in my body too high?
3. Is excess acid level in the body a cause of gout?
4. Will more alkaline food in my diet reduce the attacks of gout?

So next time you go out for a swell dinner and want to indulge yourself in good food and refreshments, think of your acid/alkaline pH level and eat fruit and vegetables to help create balance.

HAEMORRHOIDS

Haemorrhoids are definitely not glamorous. They create discomfort and are a real nuisance, as they can constantly remind the sufferer of their presence, with an annoying itch, unpleasant pain or a burning sensation. These swollen varicose veins can be internal or external and dowsing will help you to find the right treatment to remove the discomfort.

Bathing the area with Aloe Vera can be very soothing and has no side effects. Good old fashioned Witch Hazel when applied to the veins will shrink them. I am told this amazing liquid will also shrink bags under the eyes!

The plant Horse Chestnut is anti-haemorrhoid and is beneficial to this complaint and also to ulcers.

Ispaghula husk consists of natural fibre and alleviates constipation, which can aggravate the haemorrhoids. Yarrow is another old fashioned treatment which gives relief to many aches and pains.

Lady's Mantle – this little plant grows wild in fields and gardens. Soak large leaves to make an infusion and when cooled, bathe the veins with the tea. Dowse the plant Figwort, which is another old fashioned treatment. Most plant medicine is available from health shops or herbalists.

Therapists have found that the base chakra of some sufferers of haemorrhoids is out of balance. The pendulum can be used to balance this chakra.

Dowse the following:

1. Can bathing with Witch Hazel shrink the haemorrhoids?
2. Will bathing with Aloe Vera give soothing relief to this area?
3. Ask if Horse Chestnut will improve this condition?
4. Will Ispaghula husk ease the discomfort from the haemorrhoids?
5. Ask the pendulum if an infusion of Yarrow will benefit the swollen veins?
6. Is the sufferer's base chakra out of balance?

Your pendulum will confirm which of these treatments will benefit your symptoms and a good tip is to remember to avoid hot baths, as the hot water draws out the veins.

There are many old wives tales relating to illnesses and I am told that regularly massaging the heels for a few minutes each day will relieve the problem, so perhaps you would like to try this. Often it is the simplest treatment that works!

HAIR LOSS

Are you concerned that you are losing too much hair? Does your hair seem to be falling out every time you shampoo it? This problem can be caused by excess stress in your life or a shortage of certain vitamins or minerals. Dowse and ask the following:

1. Is the hair loss caused by lack of Sulphur?
2. Is your body short of Iron?
3. Is your body short of Vitamin B12?
4. Would a supplement of the amino acid Lysine stop the hair loss?
5. Essential Fatty Acids are also beneficial to hair, so check if your body would benefit from a supplement of fish oils?
6. Does your body have a Zinc deficiency? Lack of Zinc can be a cause of hair loss.

Your pendulum will help you find a natural cure for hair loss.

HEART

Heart – Arteries – Emphysema

Emphysema is a frustrating illness as it restricts your activities and there may seem to be no improvement in sight. However, don't despair! At last it looks as though there could be light at the end of the tunnel for sufferers. Results of trials showed that patients involved in the trial could walk double the distance within four weeks of taking the MSM Organic Sulphur.[1] These results are spectacular as this is a stubborn illness which often refuses to go away.

Pomegranate juice contains anti oxidants which could reduce plaque on the artery walls, so dowse and ask if this delicious juice could benefit your heart's health?

Heart – Coronary

Coronary Heart Disease can affect either young or old and is a leading cause of death in the UK. Statistics from the National Heart Forum quote that this killer illness claims the life of one in every four men and one in every six women. This heart disease is caused when the coronaries arteries become narrow due to plaque and blood flow is decreased.[6]

We hear a lot about the health benefits of Omega 3 fatty acids and rightly so as they have the ability to play a very important part in human nutrition. Omega 3 protects the heart against cardiovascular disease.

Guidelines from the American Heart Association recommend the use of fish oil and more information can be found in the British Medical Journal.[2]

Researchers now firmly believe that alpha-linolenic and ALA, one of the Omega 3's, is helpful in protecting the body against heart and vessel disease and also in lowering cholesterol levels. If you suffer from a heart problem, dowse and ask if your heart would benefit from a supplement of Omega 3?[7]

There are many natural supplements which can improve the health of the heart, so dowse and ask which of the following supplements would be beneficial. Ask your pendulum the following questions:

1. Can a supplement of Cat's Claw stop clots forming?
2. Can the correct level of Magnesium in my body help to reduces the number of attacks?
3. Does the amino acid L'Carnitine help support the heart?
4. The plant Hawthorn has been shown in German research to increase the flow of blood to the heart. Is this correct?
5. Can Red Wine or Grape Juice reduce Red platelets in the blood?
6. Is a Folic Acid deficiency a cause of many heart problems?
7. Can Digitalis from the Foxglove flower help to regulate the pulse?
8. Is Fish Oil good for the heart? Eskimo's have a diet high in fish oil and do not suffer heart problems.
9. Does Gingko Biloba ease the working of the heart?
10. Is Vitamin B6 able to prevent tiny clots which can cause arterial damage?

11. Is Vanadium able to assist the body in healing cardio-vascular illness?
12. Can the Amino Acid Lisine strip plaque from blocked arteries?
13. Ask your pendulum if your body is short of Copper, as many sufferers have a deficiency of copper.
14. Dowsing will confirm how many of the above supplements will benefit your heart problem, and the period of time they are required. You will find that several will be beneficial as they work on specific problems in the heart.

When you suspect you may have a heart problem, it is possible to dowse and establish the location of the problem. Perhaps you are suffering from Arterial Disease? If so, dowse and ask if your body is short of Chromium, as a shortage is often linked to this illness.

Sufferers of Irregular Heartbeat often have a presence of heavy metal in their blood, so check with the pendulum to ask if they have amalgam, mercury, cadmium or other heavy metals in the blood.

If you receive a 'Yes' answer, you can ask the pendulum to remove them by swinging it and asking it to show you the 'Yes' sign when it has finished the task. It may take a few minutes but it is worth attempting to remove these unwelcome contents as their presence can damage health.

Whatever the heart problem, it can be helped by balancing the heart chakra which is an important part of the body's chakra system. Dowse and ask if the heart chakra is out of balance. If you receive a 'Yes' answer, then swing the pendulum and ask it to please balance this chakra and show you the 'Yes' sign when it is balanced.

The heart has four valves: the aortic, tricupsid, mitral and pulmonary. It also has chambers, the atria and the ventricles, and two main arteries – the Coronary and the Aorta. If you have little warning signs which suggest you may have a possible heart problem you should visit your doctor, but you can also use the pendulum to confirm if there is a problem. You can dowse to check if the heart valves are all in good working order and if the arteries and the chambers are functioning correctly.

A recent study in the US involved 684 men who had suffered a heart attack and 742 men who had not suffered a heart attack. The study showed interesting results. Those who had suffered a heart attack had a 15% higher level of mercury in their blood than those men who had not suffered an attack.[4] We know that regularly eating fish which is rich in Omega 3 fatty acid is good for our health, but what happens when the fish contains mercury? Dowse and ask if your body has excess mercury?

Do you suspect that you may have a heart problem? If so, it's important to know if your mitochondrial are functioning properly. According to US cardiovascular surgeon Stephen T. Sinatra, a malfunction of the mitochondrial (*these are little batteries found in every cell*) are the cause of at least half of all patients' cardiac problems. Dowse and ask if your mitochondrial are functioning correctly? Then ask if your heart problem is linked to a mitochondrial problem?

Researchers now firmly believe that alpha-linolenic and AHA, one of the Omega 3's, is helpful in protecting the body against heart and vessel disease.

Looking after your heart is important and your pendulum will give you answers to some of the questions concerning your heart problem.

Trans Fats should be avoided in your diet when possible as these stealth killers are lurking in many foods in your larder, fridge and freezer. So what damage can these fats do to your health?

A USA Harvard School of Public Health study showed that between 30,000 and 100,000 citizens in the US die prematurely due to Trans Fats in their diet. That's a pretty awful statistic and in the UK a similar percentage of people will die from heart attacks brought on by Trans Fats in their diet.

When you add on the folks who've developed Alzheimer's disease, Type 2 Diabetes and other debilitating life threatening conditions, also linked to consumption of these Trans Fats, is it any wonder that this ingredient is restricted in Denmark? New York introduced a ban in the city's food restaurants and

Canada is considering introducing a ban. In the UK, talks are underway to introduce a ban on this killer fat and Euro MEP's have declared war on Trans Fats, demanding clear labelling of all goods containing this ingredient.

The Scotland on Sunday newspaper has opened fire on this harmful fat and reports that in the UK talks are underway with the Dept. of Health and the Food Standard Agency. Until a ban is introduced, keep dowsing your food for this hidden killer.

Although Trans Fats are on the way out, they are still on sale in a wide range of foods. In supermarkets you'll find roughly 40 products containing these fats. These killers hide in margarine, vegetable shortening, ready made pies, ice cream, puddings, potato chips, pizza, biscuits, doughnuts, gravy and sauce mixes as well as confectionary and food and sweets for children. These ingredients can be listed as hydrogenated vegetable oil, vegetable shortening or margarine and the US Food and Drug Administration's website advises you to avoid these goods.

Trans Fats are used as a cheap bulking agent, or in processed food with a long shelf life.[8]

1. Dowse and ask if regularly eating Trans Fats in your diet can affect your heart?
2. Now ask if regularly eating Trans Fats can damage your health?
3. Dowse and ask if any food in your larder contains Trans Fats?
4. Then dowse and ask if any food in your fridge contains Trans Fats?
5. Finally ask if any food in your freezer contains Trans Fats?

The message is this: 'Look after your heart – avoid Trans Fats.'

HERPES

Herpes is the Simplex virus. It's an illness that can affect anyone, even healthy individuals, so what can you do to help clear up this problem?

There are natural treatments which have been proved effective. Lemon Balm has been shown in German research to effectively treat early signs of this virus within 6 to 8 days. The Green/White Hellibore root is thought to kill this virus and amino acids Lysine and Arginine correct the balance in the body.

Another alternative is to squeeze the contents of a Vitamin E capsule on the infected spot, or try a supplement of Zinc, Kelp or Vitamin C. A course of Lithium may also help. It's time to get the pendulum out and dowse to ask if any of the above treatments will reduce your symptoms!

References

1. Regenerative Nutrition. MSM. http://www.regenerativenutrition.com Tel. 0845 034 5139. The Avenue House Developments, Sark, Channel Islands GY9 0SB UK.
2. Dr Joseph Mercola. 'How Fish Oil Protects Your Heart'. British Medical Journal 2004; 328: 30–35 Jan. 3rd 2004. www.mercola.com
3. Dr Joseph Mercola 'Are You Eating Fish Raised in Sewage?' WorldNetDay. June 4th 2007.
4. The New England Journal of Medicine Nov. 28th 2002. 347, 1735, 1736, 1747–1754, 1755–1760. Dr Joseph Mercola 'Heart Disease Linked to Mercury Contained in Fish'. www.mercola.com
5. Green Health Watch Magazine. www.greenhealthwatch.com ME CFS – Let Down by Faulty Batteries(12467) Dr Sarah Myhill.
6. National Heart Forum. www.heartforum.org.uk Coronary Heart Disease.
7. Sustainable Life. www.suslife.com 'EPA's Polyunsaturated Essential Fatty Acids – Essential to Health'.
8. TFX The Campaign Against Trans Fats. 'Trans Fats – Stealth Killers'. http://www.tfx.org
Brian Brady, Westminster Editor. Scotland on Sunday. 'Killer Fats to be Banned from Food'.
9. The World Health Organization. Fact Sheet 165. Feb. 2001. Epilepsy. Aetiogy, Epidemiology and Prognosis.
10. The World Health Organization March 2007. Sheet No. 237. 'Food Safety and Foodbourne Illness'.
11. The World Health Organization Fact Sheet No. 102 Lymphatic Filariasis.
12. The World Health Organization Fact Sheet No. 139. April 2005.
13. Food Standard Agency, 'Food Bugs' http://www.eatwell.gov.uk

14. WashingtonPost.com Tues. 7th August 2007. 'Sweet Honey', 'Could Honey, an Ancient Remedy, Make a Comeback in Contemporary Wound Care?'
15. Dr Joseph Mercola, 'A New Discovery – Gene Theory Flawed'. www.mercola.com
16. Dr Joseph Mercola 'Alaem Over Gender Bender Chemicals in Household Cleaning Products'. June 2007.
17. 'MRSA Methicillin Resistant Staphylococcus Aureus. Nexus New Times Vol. 11. No. 2. The Independent UK. Dec. 2003.
18. Center for Food Safety 'USAD Approves Application to Grow Rice With Human Genes on 270 Acres of North Carolina, Missouri'. http://www.centerforfoodsafety.org
19. Rolf Gordon, *Are you Sleeping in a Safe Place.* Available from Dulwich Health Society, 130 Gipsy Hill, London SE19 1PL. Kathe Bachler, *Earth Radiation, The Startling Discoveries of a Dowser,* Wordmaster 1989
20. Gustav Freiherr von Pohl, *Earth Currents, Causative Factor of Cancer and Other Diseases.* 1983. Published by Frech-Verlag.
21. 'Negative Ions Wipe Out Hospital Infection' Nexus, March 2003.

IATROGENIC DISEASE

Iatrogenic disease, which I mentioned briefly in the Introduction chapter, is the name they put on the death certificate when death is caused by medical error or adverse reaction to medical treatment. We don't hear much about this cause of death but it certainly appears to claim an enormous number of lives. Are we much better off and healthier taking plant medicine?

Dr Mercola reports that each year, 41,000 seniors in the USA are hospitalised for ulcers caused by medication and 32,000 suffer hip fractures attributed to drug induced falls linked to sleeping tablets or antidepressants. Gary Null's enlightening report 'Death by Medicine' tells us what some of us already suspect — that we are much healthier avoiding pharmaceutical drugs![40]

Figures from reliable sources have made surprising reading. In 2000, JAMA reported a total of 225,000 cases of Iatrogenic disease in one year. This staggering figure included medication error, hospital error and adverse effects of medication.[38]

Iatrogenic Disease is not solely a problem in the West as it also makes news in Australia. In one year, 16% of hospital deaths were from doctor or hospital error.

These figures are the result of the world's first survey into hospital safety, which was commissioned by the Australian Department of Health. The survey found that in one year, 14,000 patients died in hospital due to error and a further 30,000 suffered permanent injury.[39]

Most of us will find that these are pretty mind boggling facts. It's difficult to absorb the full extent of this information. If you are concerned about the effect of medical treatment you can dowse and ask if your illness was caused by medical error.

INFERTILITY

Dowsing female infertility problems

We are all aware of the alarming increase in the number of couples worldwide who are victims of infertility. Unfortunately, there is no set recipe for success when it comes to conceiving a baby. Fertility is a bit of a 'hit and miss' affair and can involve several factors including the right timing, health, environment etc.

This chapter is written to help couples who have experienced delays and difficulties trying to start their family.

Sometimes the problem can be serious and require medical assistance, but often the answer can be something as simple as moving your bed off a negative energy line or taking a course of a plant medicine.

There are many reasons why some women have difficulty conceiving a baby. A recent study has shown that soya should be avoided during ovulation time, as a compound in soya called genistein can sabotage the sperm as it swims towards the egg. Professor Lynn Fraser at Kings College, London told a European Fertility Conference that avoiding soya at the woman's most fertile time may aid conception.[11] This is another tip to add to the many pieces of advice given when trying to conceive.

Most of us realise that smoking cigarettes is not good for our health, particularly when pregnant, but are you aware that if you smoke when pregnant you can transmit a carcinogen to the unborn baby? This is not a warning from a bigoted non-smoker, this is fact! Research at the University of Minnesota Cancer Center analysed the first urine samples from 48 babies in a blind trial and one of the strongest carcinogens in tobacco smoke, NKK, was present in 71% of these samples. Some smokers may say that the carcinogen could have come from food or any other source, but the carcinogen NKK is only found in tobacco and was not found in the urine of babies whose mothers were non-smokers.

Dowse and ask your pendulum if the carcinogen NKK can be passed from the mother to the foetus?

Now ask your pendulum if the carcinogen NKK can travel to the foetus simply by the mother regularly being present in a room with tobacco smoke?

As well as possibly damaging the health of the unborn baby, research has shown tobacco smoke can increase the risk of Cot

Deaths. Swedish research autopsy results showed that of 24 SID deaths, all but two babies had nicotine contained in their lungs.[34] Dowse and ask your pendulum if smoking tobacco during pregnancy increases the risk of Cot Death?

Tips to help you conceive

Dowse and ask your pendulum if any of the following tips will help to enable you to conceive.

1. Stop smoking.
2. Reduce alcohol intake – it can inhibit ovulation, affect sperm transformation and possibly affect estrogen receptors in the liver.
3. Eat plenty fruit and vegetables to build up the alkaline level.
4. Don't use a sun bed or electric blanket.
5. Stop taking the pill three months before you plan to conceive to allow the body to adjust.
6. Lie still for 30 minutes after sex to help the sperm have a smooth journey to the egg.
7. Don't use a lubricant as this can kill the sperm.
8. Leave the penis in the vagina until limp to stop semen leak.
9. Place a pillow under your bottom before sex to tip the pelvis.
10. Don't urinate, wash or douche immediately after love making.

Apologies for the simplicity of the above list. Some are perhaps very obvious tips, and some of them you have probably already tried or been told about, but remember it is often the simplest things that work – ask your pendulum to check the list.

Some natural causes of infertility

Infertility can often be caused by certain glands in the body being out of balance, or perhaps the ovaries need healing. Start by asking your pendulum if your infertility is caused by an imbalance in a gland or a mineral deficiency? If you have been 'on the Pill' for several years, there is a possibility that your body could be short of Copper and B vitamins. Candida is also common after the Pill, so these are all questions you can dowse.

1. Ask your pendulum if your ovaries would benefit from receiving a session of Healing? You can use the pendulum to send healing energy to the ovaries.
2. Dowse each of the following glands separately, asking if they are correctly balanced? Also, ask if there are any blockages in the glands?

(1) Hypothalamus, (2) Pituitary, (3) Thyroid, (4) Endocrine, (5) Adrenal and (6) Sex Glands?

There are so many different factors which can cause infertility. These can include certain glands being out of balance, so cleanse your pendulum and then start by asking the question 'Are all of these glands balanced?' then ask 'Are there any blockages in any of these glands?'

If you receive a 'Yes' answer, you can then dowse each gland individually to find which glands are out of balance, and which have energy blockages.

You can then use your pendulum to balance the glands and to remove the blockages. Now ask your pendulum if the Pancreatic enzyme function is correct? Does the body have excess heavy metals?

Some women who have been unable to conceive a baby have found that once the Geopathic Stress has been removed, they then conceive.

Miscarriages as well as infertility can be caused by exposure to certain chemicals. Time magazine reported pregnant mothers working in silicon chip production were exposed to two solvent chemicals and the rate of miscarriages amongst this group of women was double the normal figure.[5(e)]

If your pendulum has still not located the cause of the infertility, dowse and ask the following questions:

1. Is there an imperfection in my pelvis?

2. Do I have a cervical infection?
3. Am I failing to ovulate?
4. Is there a blockage in the Fallopian tubes?
5. Are there ovarian problems?
6. Unhealthy sperm?

These are all questions you can ask your pendulum before you consult a doctor, as some of the problems can be resolved with the aid of the pendulum.

As I mentioned earlier, if you have been on the pill, you may have a Copper deficiency. As Copper enhances fertility and is needed to release the Luteinizing hormone produced by the Hypothalamus, it is important to check that the body has the correct level of this mineral.

As well as Copper, there are many other vitamins and minerals you can be short of in your diet that play an important role in good health and fertility. Dowse and ask your pendulum if your body is short of any of the following listed below and then ask if your body would benefit from a supplement of any of them.

Copper, Kelp, Lecithin, Ginseng, Brewers Yeast, Manganese, Molybdenum, Choline, Inositol, Calcium, Magnesium, Vitamins A, B, C, E and the plants Feverfew and Agnus Caster (*a hormone regulator*).

It's now time to check the energy balance of certain areas of the body which can affect fertility, so dowse and ask if each one is balanced.

1. Is my Conception Meridian clear?
2. Is the Estrogen/Progesterone level balanced?
3. Are my body's 7 main chakras balanced?
4. Does my body have an overload of toxins?

Hormone imbalance can be rectified with the help of plant Estrogen, so if your pendulum has confirmed that your Estrogen/Progesterone level is wrong, you can dowse the following plants which are known to help regulate this problem. Firstly ask if a supplement of any of the following plants will be beneficial and if you receive a 'Yes' answer you can dowse each one individually. (1) Wild Yam, (2) Alfalfa, (3) Celery, (4) Ginseng, (5) Fennel, or (6) Rhubarb.

Pelvic inflammatory disease

Female infertility can often be caused by damage to the Fallopian tubes, which can occur due to any of the following causes. Dowse and ask if any of them are linked to your fertility problem.

1. Adhesions from abdominal or pelvic surgery?
2. Endometriosis?
3. Colitis?
4. Ectopic pregnancy?

Pelvic inflammatory disease includes high temperature, pain in the pelvic area, vaginal discharge, low back pain or pain when love making. These symptoms can be caused by any of the following conditions, so you can dowse to find the cause.

1. Infection from removal of a coil?
2. Infection after birth, miscarriage or abortion?
3. Are you suffering from a sexually transmitted disease?

Next, I have listed a selection of supplements and treatments, so dowse to find which will be beneficial for your health.

Dowse the plants Echinacea, Golden Seal and Rosemary. Ask your pendulum if Tea Tree oil in bath water would reduce the inflammation? Would a massage with Clary Sage oil be beneficial? This oil is known to act directly on the ovaries to restore low estrogen. Your pendulum will point you in the direction of the most helpful treatment.

Irregular periods

Another problem which affects fertility is suffering irregular periods. Here are a few tips which may help to resolve this problem, whether you are trying to conceive or not.

Liquorice is known to help regulate the menstrual cycle and improve ovulation. The Agnes Castus plant, as I mentioned earlier, regulates hormones and is a good friend to all women. The homeopathic remedy Sepia is beneficial, and Ginseng and Dong Qua are also known to help resolve hormone problems.

Painful periods

Painful periods can be a real nightmare to many women, as they can disrupt life and work for several days each month by causing dreadful pain. Dowse and ask if any of the following will help resolve your period problem:

1. Are you sleeping over Geopathic Stress?
2. Is the problem caused by a mineral or vitamin deficiency?
3. Would a supplement of B6 and also B Complex be beneficial?
4. Would any of the following help to resolve the problem?

Dowse and ask separately – (1) Magnesium, (2) Zinc, (3) Iron, (4) Feverfew, (5) Black Haw.

It is now time to talk about miscarriages – what can cause them and how, when possible, to avoid them.

Miscarriage

There is a wide variety of possible causes of a miscarriage and each situation can be very different, so here are a few possible causes to dowse.

1. A Blood Clotting Disorder?
2. A Chromosome imbalance? (*Chromosomes carry genetic information.*)
3. Polycystic Ovaries? (*This is found in a high percentage of women who miscarry.*)
4. Disruption of Antibodies?
5. Abnormalities of the Womb?

Whatever the cause of a miscarriage, it is important to consult a doctor.

What The Doctors Don't Tell You Magazine published an article on research results of the effect of cough mixtures on chicken embryos.

Most Cough mixtures contain Dextromethorphan, which is so powerful that one dose has been found to be a possible cause of birth defects and miscarriages.[35]

When you have suffered a miscarriage, your body is often depleted in energy and needs supplements to help you regain good health. Dowse and ask if your body would benefit from a supplement of Multi Minerals, Essential fatty acids, Feverfew, Manganese, Selenium, Ginseng, Magnesium or Copper. Dowse each one individually.

Can infertility and miscarriages be linked to chemicals and pesticide exposure?

Immune system imbalance can be linked to some cases of miscarriages and infertility. This occurs when autoimmune antibodies revolt (the antibodies mistakenly attack the person's body). Research shows this situation occurs in 33% of women who miscarry. This research from Tel Aviv showed that in the control group, women who had successful pregnancies all had 0% of autoimmune antibodies present in their body.[5(d)]

A Canadian research project found 20% to 25% of miscarriages are due to the immune system being low, which confirms results of the Tel Aviv research. [5(f)]

Geopathic stress

I have cleared Geopathic Stress from the homes of a number of women who have had several unexplained miscarriages and were sleeping over Geopathic Stress energy. GS can lower the immune system of an individual, making it harder to fight those dangerous antibodies. This situation is very common and many women find that after this negative energy had been cleared from their home, they are often able to carry a baby to full term. Also, some women who have been unable to conceive a baby have found that once the Geopathic Stress has been removed, they then conceive. It is very important to dowse to check that you are not sleeping or working over Geopathic Stress. If the pendulum gives a positive answer, then it's time to ask the pendulum to remove the Geopathic Stress and show you the 'Yes' sign when it is cleared.

Male infertility problems

Male infertility on today's scale is a modern day problem which affects men in all walks of life in many countries. Alas, the Male sperm is not what it used to be! It's official – a report from the Institute of Environmental Health Science, a federal agency, states that serious deterioration of the male reproductive system is affecting males in many parts of the world. This government agency suggests the root cause may be environmental chemicals interfering with male hormones.[3(a)] Yes, this is one of the many problems facing today's male sperm, but there are several other threats. Dowsing will help to diagnose the cause of each person's problem.

The report describes negative trends in male reproductive health, confirms similar findings among wildlife and tells us that these problems being experienced in the US have also been experienced in Europe since the early 90's.

As well as reporting on the increase in infertility problems, the report advises us there has been a noticeable increase in the incidence of Hyposadias (a birth defect of the penis) and Cryptochidism (undescended testicles).[3]

If you or any friend or family member suffering from any of these problems, you can dowse the questions:

1. Is Hyposadias linked to unnatural toxic chemicals in the body?
2. Is Cryptochidism linked to exposure to certain toxic chemicals?
3. Are a percentage of reproductive problems linked to toxic chemicals in the body?
4. Are a number of cases of infertility linked to exposure to certain toxic chemicals

In the UK alone, roughly 2.5 million men are affected by this distressing and frustrating problem. This number of sufferers seems ridiculously high, but these figures are reported by Norwich Union Healthcare[10], so are not a piece of sensational journalism! We are talking about 9% of males, which suggests that an alarming number of couples will be affected. The long term implications of these figures paint a bleak picture.

Sperm count is a sensitive area and can very easily be affected by conditions either inside or outside of the body. Low sperm count is the most common cause of infertility, but infertility can also be caused by low sperm mobility, lack of semen or due to bad quality of sperm. So what is the most likely cause of these infertility problems which seem increasingly common in men from different careers and backgrounds?

Dowse and ask your pendulum the following questions:

1. Is my sperm count low?
2. Is my low sperm count caused by low sperm mobility?
3. Is the low sperm count caused by lack of semen?
4. Is it caused by bad quality of the semen?

Do you enjoy long soaks in the steam tub or regularly indulge in a relaxing sauna? The bad news is that some cases of low sperm count are linked to lifestyle. Several well known situations, like overheating from taking regular saunas or steam tubs, can disrupt this sensitive mechanism. Are you a cycling enthusiast? Mountain biking, cycle racing and triathlon racing are increasing in popularity amongst energetic young males and research suggests that the pressure of the cycle's seat creates erectile dysfunction, although this factor would only affect a small number of males.[1]

The Journal of Sexual Medicine reports three studies on the effects of bike riding and the male reproductive system. Health researcher Steven Schrader's report on police officers showed that biking officers experienced more problems than non-biking officers. Again, only a small number of men are affected by this cause, so what is the most common cause of infertility?[2]

Dowse and ask the following questions:

1. Does a regular soak in the steam tub have an adverse effect on my sperm count?
2. Does a regular leisurely sauna have an adverse effect on my sperm count?

Stress at work and at home can be a cause of low sperm count and some scientists believe laptop computer use can be responsible for a few cases of infertility, as laptop computers give off heat and, as I mentioned earlier, heat is detrimental to sperm count. They are also invariably used on the male lap, close to the genital area of the body.

As well as giving off heat, these clever gadgets give off electromagnetic energy which can affect the body's energy field. Laptops are still an unknown quantity.

Dowse and ask if your sperm count is aggravated by any of the following:

1. Stress at work?
2. Excess alcohol?
3. Use of recreational drugs?
4. Your laptop computer regularly used on your lap?
5. Your mobile phone in your trouser pocket?

Are disposable nappies a fertility threat?

You've probably heard some mothers mention their concern that using disposable nappies could affect their baby's fertility. This is entirely possible, as it's an accepted fact that the male genitals should not be overheated due to the affect on sperm count. A German study 'The Archives of Disease in Childhood,' found that a baby's disposable nappy is capable of raising the temperature to one degree above natural body heat and showed that the disposable nappy impaired the body's natural testicular cooling mechanism.[9]

Most babies and toddlers wear a nappy for the first two years of their life. Does receiving constant heat in their genitals for this length of time cause long term damage to their reproductive organs? The heat plus chemicals from the plastic liner and plastic pants are not a good combination.

Come back terry nappies! I well remember the never ending washing of terry nappies and trying to get them dry in winter weather, so I acknowledge the convenience of disposable nappies, but quite apart from the possible health damage they may cause, they are not planet friendly.

Mothers who opt to avoid using disposable nappies due to their concern over fertility effects are certainly doing planet Earth a big favour, as disposable nappies are a landfill's nightmare!

Dowse the following:

1. Can disposable nappies cause your child's genitals to overheat?
2. You can then dowse several brands, asking which is least harmful. You can complete this exercise by writing a list of well-known brands and then dowsing each one separately.
3. You can also dowse to ask if Terry toweling nappies would be more beneficial for your child's health.

Chemicals and damage to the male sperm

Research has been carried out in many countries on infertility linked to exposure to certain chemicals and many results suggest that by far the biggest damaging influence on male sperm comes from certain chemicals and pesticides. The source of exposure to these chemicals can be extremely varied, ranging from the foetus absorbing toxic chemicals from the mother while still cosy in the womb, to being accidentally sprayed by pesticide. Most of us don't think of possibilities such as contaminated water when looking for a cause for infertility, but it's essential to explore every avenue.

News is reaching the media that the chemical compound Bisphenyl A (BPA) is in big trouble. Several dozen scientists have issued a very strong warning that this estrogen-like compound in plastics, which is one of the highest volume plastics in the world, is known to be a likely cause of several serious reproductive disorders and has found its way into the human body.

Five separate new reviews, plus a new study by the National Institute of Health which summarised 700 studies, all suggest that this chemical compound is not good for human health. The scientists concluded that the animal research showed female reproductive problems, tract disorders, breast and prostate cancer and a decreased level of sperm count.[17] As decreased sperm count is already a serious problem, we certainly don't need any possible reproductive toxic chemicals in our bodies increasing this problem. Dr Joseph Mercola warns us that it is difficult to avoid this compound, as it's already in the atmosphere and in our water.

A thought which greatly concerns me is that if baby's bottles contain this chemical compound, does it stay in their body for many years? Will it affect their reproductive system in years to come?

Dowse and ask the following questions:

1. Can the chemical compound BisphenylA (BPA) in the plastic in babies bottles leech to the baby?
2. Can the chemical compound Bisphenyl A (BPA) damage human health?
3. Can this chemical leech from the linings of cans to the food?
4. Can the chemical mimic the hormone Estradoil?

Bisphenyl A (BPA) is used in the manufacture of hard plastic items including can food liners, microwave oven food dishes, sports bottles, polycarbonate plastic baby bottles and some dental sealants for children.

Another form of chemical contamination can be caused by chemicals in pesticides used in the farming of fields nearby draining into water supplies, or a thoughtless person dumping unwanted chemicals into a local stream.

A correct balance of the natural hormones in the body is vital to enable the reproductive process to work smoothly. This sensitive mechanism is easily disrupted by the presence of foreign, unnatural chemicals. Perhaps the worst disrupters are chemicals which mimic the natural estrogens and create infertility problems by thoroughly confusing the body's estrogen receptors. Among the offending chemicals are a variety of plastics including PVC, petroleum based products, PCB's and Dioxins.[5]

Copenhagen gives us more confirmation that sperm count is reducing in healthy males; Danish scientists report that sperm has dropped over a fifty year period. This suggests that the average male now produces less than half as many sperm as were produced by men half a century ago.[6(a)] BBC News recently reported that studies from Denmark, France and Argentina all confirmed a decline in this important body function. Even worse, researchers found that those men who had been exposed to pesticides, as well as suffering low sperm count also had higher levels of two female sex hormones in their system, compared with men who had not been in contact with pesticides.

It is so important to be aware of the possible danger to sperm from chemicals. Reliable research has shown they are a hidden enemy to men in all age groups.[12]

Dowse and ask the following:

1. Is drinking water in your workplace contaminated with chemicals?
2. Is drinking water in my home contaminated with chemicals?
3. Are there any Dioxins my drinking water?

We know that the presence of chemicals mimicking the body's estrogen is a serious problem but in addition to this, some of these environmental chemicals have been shown in laboratory animals to have a long half life and can bio-accumulate as a result.[6(b)] Exposure to high levels of two hormone disrupting organo-chlorine pesticides (Vinclozolin and Methoxychlor) while in the womb can cause infertility problems up to four generations later. This incredibly upsetting fact was unveiled in a new study published in the June 3rd 2005 issue of the Journal *Science* by Michael Skinner PhD, and his team at Washington State University.

The implications of these facts paint a very gloomy picture for the next four generations and call for drastic action to redress this problem which affects so many families and has already spiralled out of control.[12]

Convincing proof that in some cases living in the country can affect fertility comes from research in the US. The research showed that sperm count in rural workers in Missouri was 42% lower than men living in urban Minneapolis. During the research, urine was checked for the breakdown products of 15 different farm chemicals. Results published in Environmental Health Perspectives showed that the men with high levels of the herbicide Alachlor in their systems were 30 times more likely to have diminished sperm quality.[7]

This research by Shannah H. Swan and her team of researchers shows poor semen quality is often associated with high levels of certain chemicals found in the urine.[15] If you are experiencing infertility problems, perhaps it's time to have your urine checked for the presence of chemicals.

Infertility in women living in farmland areas has been shown in many cases to be linked to exposure to herbicides and fungicides. Results of a recent study published in the Epidemiology show that infertile women who live near US farmland were 27 times more likely to have used fungicides within the two years prior to their infertility problems developing.[13] Just in case exposure to certain chemicals can disrupt your fertility, you have an excellent excuse for refusing to use herbicides on the vegetable plot until your child bearing years are over.

In this study, 1,791 potential cases were screened, along with 822 potential controls and of these, 322 cases and 322 matched controls were involved in the study.[14]

Further confirmation that pesticides are possibly one of fertility's worst enemies comes from Holland. A study involving 836 couples showed that those who had been exposed to pesticides were nearly four times less likely to have children than couples who had not been exposed to these toxins.[8]

The implications that male infertility has increased dramatically over the past few decades leaves us feeling a bit bewildered, wondering where it will all end. Dr Cecil Jacobson from the Reproductive Genetic Center in Virginia reports a 15 fold increase in the functionally sterile sector of males suffering infertility. (This is defined as sperm counts below 20 million per millilitre of sperm.)[5(a)]

Many folks wrongly assume that when a couple have difficulty conceiving a baby, the problem is usually caused by the woman having gynecological problems. Dr Pat McShane of the Department of Obstetrics & Gynecology in Boston, Massachusetts reports that 40% of all infertility cases today are due to male problems.[5(b)] There may be slight variations in the exact numbers of male sufferers, depending on the research carried out, but all confirm that there are a high number of males who will experience fertility problems.

Experts tell us that most families in the western world live in pesticide contaminated homes and, in the US, approximately 70% of homes are found to contain the pesticide chlordane.[5(c)] The presence of these unwelcome unnatural chemicals is likely to disrupt the health of any person whose immune system is slightly below par.

It's hard to believe but there are more than 70,000 synthetic or naturally occurring chemicals in commercial use today and many have not been examined for toxicity, to find how they interact with other chemicals. Dowse and ask if this figure is roughly correct?

Confirmation has come from many scientists that exposure to solvents, certain pesticides and some industrial chemicals can cause infertility and create hormonal disruption. Birth defects are also linked to exposure to these substances, which I have already mentioned, along with chromosome damage and menstrual problems.

Certain heavy metals raise cause for alarm during pregnancy or when experiencing infertility problems. These include lead, arsenic, mercury and cadmium.

Lead can cause functional defects, female infertility, hormonal disruption and low birth weight. Found in contaminated food, soil, tap water and old paint.

Arsenic can cause spontaneous abortion, structural birth defects, low birth weight and damage to hearing. It is found in contaminated water, in the atmosphere in industrial areas, in dry cleaning and industrial processes.

Formaldehyde is known to create birth abnormalities and spontaneous abortion. It is found in new carpets, industrial processes and dry cleaning chemicals.

Mercury is linked to menstrual abnormalities, spontaneous abortion and is found in dental fillings, fish, dry cleaning fluid and industrial processes.

Another 'No No' is the group of endocrine disrupters which include dioxins, PCB's, phthalates alkylphenyls and certain pesticides. The smooth functioning of the endocrine system is vital so these intruders are bad news.[22]

Mercury can affect fertility so if you are having difficulty conceiving a baby, perhaps it's time to have the Mercury level checked for you and your partner. Many Amalgam fillings leak Mercury, which is a reproductive toxin.

Dowse the following questions:

1. Do you have excess Mercury in your body?
2. Does your partner have excess Mercury in their body?
3. Are your amalgam fillings leaking Mercury?
4. Are your partner's amalgam fillings leaking Mercury?

It is hardly surprising that Mercury can affect fertility; a mere $\frac{1}{2}$ a gram can contaminate the ecosystem of a 10 acre lake to the extent that health warnings are issued not to eat the fish. This warning applies to half of the rivers and lakes in Florida and the effect is also felt in other areas. 20% of all the Great Lakes in the US have health warnings about eating fish caught there.

Dental Amalgam fillings are the largest source of Methyl Mercury in most people and those folks who have several amalgam fillings have Mercury excretion 10 times the average of those without these fillings. After the removal of Amalgam, most folks have a 90% reduction in the Mercury level in their saliva and excretion.[36]

Dowse and ask if any of the above metals or chemicals are linked to your infertility? Asking the right questions about an infertility problem will enable you to trace the cause of the problem and also find a possible remedy. As well as dowsing for causes, you can use the pendulum to confirm the time of the month at which you are most fertile and also the time at which you are the least! Dowsing is truly an invaluable tool to help couples with infertility problems, to pinpoint the source and rectify it. Remember, it is important to cleanse the pendulum and to phrase the questions in several different ways to ensure that you get the correct answer.

The researchers I have quoted do not have any financial interest in the results of their research, so are not biased when reporting the findings of their studies.

Now it's time to talk about supplements which may resolve the problem. Selenium is known to increase the sperm count so if a low count is the problem, think Selenium! The Health Guardian in February '97 reported test trials had shown an increase in sperm mobility after taking 130 micrograms of Selenium daily for three months. The trials completed 10 years ago but the problem is still the same so dowse and ask if a supplement of Selenium would improve your sperm quality?

The Amino Acid Arginine is reported to increase sperm count and overall sperm activity, so this is another avenue to explore.

Dowse and ask if a supplement of Selenium would improve the sperm problem?

Now dowse and ask if a supplement of Arginine would improve the sperm problem?

Dowse and ask separately if a supplement of any one or more on the following list would improve the sperm problem. If you receive a 'Yes' answer, Dowse each of the following plants, minerals, vitamins and amino acids. (1) L'Carnitine, (2) Lysine, (3) Arginine, (4) Saw Palmento, (5) Sarsaparillo, (6) Siberian Ginseng, (7) Yohimbe, (8) Essential Fatty Acids, (9) Kelp, (10) Chromium, (11) Liquorice root, (12) Lecithin, (13) Vitamins A, B, C and E.

You can also dowse and ask if your body has too high or too low a level of the trace mineral Vanadium. Should you receive a 'Yes' sign to either question you can ask your pendulum to please balance the level.

I now want you to check your body for some natural causes which can instigate infertility. Did you suffer from Mumps as a child? Dowse and ask if the vibration of the Mumps virus is linked to your fertility problem. Should you receive confirmation that it is one of the culprits, cleanse your pendulum and then ask it to please remove the vibration of the Mumps virus from your body.

Next, ask if the testosterone level is balanced. If the level is wrong, you can ask the pendulum to correct the balance.

Perhaps your Prostate gland is in need of healing? Or maybe there is scar tissue in the venous vein? Dowse and ask your pendulum a few questions to try and locate the problem. The Pituitary gland plays an important part in fertility so ask your pendulum if your Pituitary gland is balanced? Should you receive a 'No' answer, you can ask your pendulum to balance the gland.

A shortage of Vitamin A can damage sperm producing cells and Vitamin C is necessary for sperm motility and morbidity. Zinc also helps sperm motility and production.

Male impotence problem

Impotence can be caused by low testosterone count or diminished blood circulation to the genitals. Dowse and ask if you suffer from either of these problems?

Next, ask if your Thyroid gland is out of balance? It may be over active or under active.

Are any unwelcome parasites of fungus in your body? These uninvited guests can interfere with your sex life so if you receive a 'Yes' sign, you will find remedies in the health shop which can remove these nuisances. You could also try asking your pendulum to remove them!

Colloidal silver is an excellent treatment to remove parasites, so dowse and ask if this tasteless liquid would remove any parasites in your body? Impotence can be helped by a supplement of some of the following plants so dowse and ask if any of the following would resolve your impotence problem. If you receive a 'Yes' answer, dowse each one separately. (1) Burdock root, (2) Damiana leaves, (3) Gravel root (queen of the meadow), (4) Plantian, (5) Poke Root (pigeon berry), (6) St. John's Wort, (7) Wintergreen, (8) Fenegreek, (9) Black Walnut or (10) Kelp. The Trace mineral Vanadium can also be helpful. Dowse and ask which of these supplements will help to resolve the impotence?

Male erection problems

This problem is one which sufferers may prefer not to discuss but perhaps some tips on this page will help to resolve this frustrating problem.

When you regularly experience the disappointment of an erection which will not last then it's Arginine to the rescue. This amino acid has helped many sufferers. The homeopathic remedy Conium can also help with this difficulty. Dowse and ask if a supplement of Arginine will help resolve this difficulty? Will a supplement of the homeopathic remedy Conium will be beneficial? Yohimbe aids erection so ask your pendulum to confirm whether or not it will help you.

Do you often have an erection when you are half asleep and as soon as you are awake it wilts? Well, Caladium has helped many folks resolve this problem, so dowse and ask your pendulum if this homeopathic remedy will resolve the nuisance.

Are you regularly annoyed by an erection which is not firm enough for the job? Dowse and ask if a supplement of Arginine, Agnus Castus or Yohimbe will improve the quality of your erection.

Men who suffer from Premature Ejaculation sometimes find a supplement of multi minerals, Vitamin E, Zinc and Amino Acids resolves this common upset.

Low Sex Drive is a modern day problem which is perhaps in some cases linked to stress and working long hours. A supplement of Catuaba may be the answer as this plant from Brazil is a sexual stimulant and a tonic to the genitals. Dowse and ask if a supplement of this plant will be beneficial! Wild Yam, root and also Yahombe are all useful aids so get dowsing and hopefully you will be able to resolve your problem.

Animals and reproductive problems

It's not only we humans whose reproductive system can be upset by exposure to certain chemicals – very strange things are happening in the world of animals and sea creatures. They have become victims of pesticides and chemicals which are playing havoc with their reproductive systems.

Sadly, alligators living in pesticide contaminated lakes in Florida are experiencing severe reproduction problems. Their penises are now so small due to exposure to hormone disrupting pesticides in their natural surroundings that they have become sexually incompetent.

These alligators are not the only victims of pesticide. Turtles in Florida are finding that PCB's are playing havoc with their eggs. These are not isolated incidences; I recall hearing ten years ago that roughly 90% of the flounders in a river in the north of England were unable to reproduce as pesticides in the river had caused deformity of their sexual organs.

Animals are affected by pesticides either in their drinking water, or from eating other species contaminated with toxins. A really sad example of this is the beautiful panthers in Florida – many of them have un-descended testicles, poor sperm production and other reproductive problems due to eating raccoons who have become contaminated with these chemicals from the fish they eat. Please be warned! Pesticides seem to have succeeded in rapidly entering the animal food chain and the seriousness of

141

this situation must never be underestimated. We could be the next victims! Contamination of one species leads to contamination of another species and this may continue until it reaches the foods we humans eat![3]

Minks and river otters in the Columbia River in North America are also victims of genital abnormalities. Both species display Hypospadias, which is arrested development of the penis. The normal opening, instead of being situated on the top of the penis, is on the underside. In some extreme cases, these poor animals have been born with the hole so far back it was at the scrotum, making reproduction an impossibility. If this condition affects an increasing numbers of species, it won't be many years before they become extinct. And what about humans?

Chemical manufacturers assure us pesticides and other organo chlorine chemicals do not cause any health problems. Is it only a coincidence that these pesticides have been found in animals and shown to cause Hyposadias in laboratory animals?[6]

I have tried to cover a wide range of suggestions and possibilities linked to infertility in this chapter and I hope this information will help many folks resolve this upsetting problem.

IMMUNE SYSTEM

Autoimmune illnesses are becoming increasingly common. It makes us wonder what the explanation is for the increase in such illnesses as Chronic Fatigue Syndrome, Fibromyalgia, Crohn's Disease, Lupus, Multiple Sclerosis, Psoriasis, Rheumatic Arthritis and many more.

So what causes autoimmune illnesses? It happens when your body is not working correctly and mistakes your own cells for invaders, declaring war on them. In other words, your body attacks itself. This attack can take place in any area of the body so you may develop a problem in glands, heart, blood, joints, kidneys, lungs or the brain.

The Immune System is the body's protection system which helps the body to identify and fight illnesses and viruses.

Today, the Immune System has to work harder than ever before as there are so many environmental toxins, viruses and electromagnetic fields which weaken this important defence system. It works very hard to discourage harmful substances from entering the body and the body's own antibiotics fight any foreign invaders.

This system is a busy area of the body. It consists of an enormous number of white blood cells and antibodies as well as the bone marrow and the Thymus gland. They all work to protect us against the army of microbes which penetrate our body including harmful bacteria in food and the environment, viruses and parasites galore.

Your immune system gives you warning signs when it is low – you may feel tired and lacking in energy, or constantly catching colds and tummy bugs. It is so important to keep your immune system strong so that it is always on guard to fight any onslaught of illness.

It's hard to believe that autoimmune illnesses are caused by the body's immunological defences attacking its own tissues. As you can imagine, when the body begins behaving in this manner, it is difficult to change the pattern without knowing the cause.

This group of illnesses include Lupus, Type 1 Diabetes and Multiple Sclerosis. Lupus produces rheumatic type symptoms, causing pain in joints and other areas of the body. Type 1 Diabetes occurs when the confused immune system attacks the pancreas. In Multiple Sclerosis, it attacks the fatty sheaths of nerve cells.

So what causes the body to declare war on itself? Some folks blame fluoride, mercury or arsenic in the environment, while others say it is linked to the presence of phthalates or dioxins. If you suffer from an immune system illness, dowse to ask the cause.

1. Is my illness linked to food ingredients?
2. Has my immune system been damaged by toxic chemicals in the environment?
3. Is the illness linked to chemicals in drinking water?

Never in the history of mankind has the immune system had to contend with so many enemies. Today, it is constantly being bombarded by toxins galore, powerful electromagnetic fields and harmful chemicals in the food chain.

We also use hair, skin and bath treatments which contain chemicals that soak through the skin into our bloodstreams. The poor immune system has to work full time to combat the onslaught and is often fighting a losing battle. We see fine examples of this fact in the enormous increase of immune related illnesses including cancer, Lupus and a list of other illnesses. The big questions is 'How do we strengthen our immune system?'

Many folks swear by the plant Echinacea, which does a wonderful job of strengthening the immune system and of defending against flu and colds each winter. Germanium has been shown to quickly reduce pain and strengthen the immune system so is an excellent supplement.

Often when your immune system is low, your body is short of certain important minerals. Dowse and ask if your body would benefit from a supplement of any of the following minerals, plants or amino acids: (1) Cat's Claw, (2) Echinacea, (3) Lapacho, (4) Garlic, (5) Liquorice, (6) Iron, (7) Manganese, (8) Germanium or (9) Glutathione.

The antioxidant Selenium fights free radicals, so ask if a supplement of this mineral would be beneficial.

Heavy Metals are a real threat to the immune system so dowse and ask whether your body has an excess of any of the following: (1) Mercury, (2) Arsenic, (3) Cadmium or (4) Lead?

If you receive a 'Yes' sign for any of these health hazards then cleanse your pendulum and ask it to please remove the excess from your body.

You are probably mentally asking how you could possibly have excess heavy metals in your body, but it is quite easy to innocently acquire them. Excess mercury can come from amalgam fillings, from cooking utensils and occasionally from drinking water. If you live in an industrial area then arsenic is found in the atmosphere, and lead can be absorbed from old paintwork. These are just a few of the threats from heavy metals but it gives you an idea of the scale of this modern day health hazard.

Formaldehyde is a hidden enemy found in new carpets, so dowse and ask if your new carpets are giving off formaldehyde? If you receive a 'Yes' answer, make a point of keeping windows open at every opportunity to clear the atmosphere.

Research at Montana's Center of Environmental Health Perspectives found a link between autoimmunity and exposure to Asbestos. Researchers found that the group of residents involved in the research, who all lived in a small town in Montana which was polluted with Asbestos, had a 28% higher level of harmful autoimmunities in their blood than the group who lived in a town free from asbestos pollution.

There are many causes of this group of illnesses and asbestos is one more to add to the list of hazards. If you live in an industrial area where Asbestos is in the environment, or even if you live in a small village where Asbestos was used in buildings, perhaps you would like to dowse to ask if Asbestos is the cause of your illness?[30]

Chemicals can enter our body from so many innocent looking products, particularly beauty creams, hair products and bath lotions. Dowse each of the products you use regularly and ask if they contain any chemicals which are harmful to your health? Ask if any of these chemicals soak through your skin into your blood stream? If you are alarmed about this effect on your health and want to purchase chemical free products, there is an abundance of them available in health shops due to the increasing number of people becoming aware of this health hazard and turning to chemical free products.

Is your illness possibly linked to an imbalance of acid/alkaline pH? So many of us eat food which is mainly acid forming and neglect to eat alkaline foods, so dowse and ask if your symptoms will improve if you include more alkaline food in your diet. Get into the habit of eating green vegetables and fruit, as they will help to balance the pH in your body. Dowse and ask if your body's acid/alkaline level is correct?

Finally, the greatest enemy of the immune system is Geopathic Stress. If you are unfortunate enough to be sleeping or working over GS, your immune system is being bombarded with negative energy every night as you sleep or each day as you sit at your desk. You may suspect your immune system is low if perhaps you waken each morning feeling tired, or you seem to get one cold or bug after another. Dowse and check if you are being exposed to these powerful negative rays? If you receive a 'Yes' answer then, first, cleanse your pendulum. Next, ask it to please remove the Geopathic Stress from the building and show you the 'yes' sign when this has been carried out. The job may take a few minutes, so relax and know your immune system will benefit greatly from this simple task.

'*Good news for all sufferers of Autoimmune illnesses.*' The US National Institute of Health (NIH) has awarded $51 million dollars to expand research on this group of illnesses. The American Autoimmune Related Diseases Association reports that there are 89 separate, clinically distinct autoimmune diseases and between 14 and 22 million sufferers in the US, and many millions more in other countries.[29]

INCONTINENCE

Incontinence is an embarrassing problem which can affect any one of us and sufferers don't tend to mention their problem. One possible cause is fluoride in toothpaste. Dowse and ask if your incontinence problem is caused by using toothpaste containing fluoride?

Below I have listed a few helpful suggestions, so please dowse and ask if any of these would improve your condition. If you receive a 'Yes' answer, please dowse each one separately.

1. Dowse and ask if Saw Palmetto would heal a leaky bladder?
2. Would DHEA hormone help the leaky bladder?
3. Will Cranberry Juice improve my Bladder problem?
4. Will Echinacea reduce inflammation in the bladder?
5. Bearberry is thought to strengthen the sphincter muscle to resolve leaky bladder problems, so ask if it will help you.

Dowsing can often help sufferers to find a natural, pain-free treatment to end incontinence.

INSOMNIA

Most of us spend approximately one third of our life asleep in bed, which is beneficial – a good pattern of sleep is essential for good health. Lack of sleep can create all sorts of health problems, including lack of concentration and irritability, while insomnia can ruin your quality of life. Finding the cause of disturbed sleep is therefore very important. After that, the next step is to find a non-addictive treatment free of side effects. This is when dowsing is an invaluable tool!

There are so many different factors which can cause disruption of your sleep pattern and create a serious Insomnia nightmare. As the reasons are so varied, before treating the problem it is important to find the source to enable you to break the pattern. Dowse the following questions:

1. Is your insomnia caused by stress either at home or work?
2. Is it caused by worry over a family member?
3. Is it caused by financial worries?
4. Is it caused by job worries?
5. Is it caused by sleeping over Geopathic Stress?
6. Is your sleep problem caused by a shortage of melatonin in your body?
7. Is bad Feng Shui linked to your sleep problem?
8. Is negative energy from outside your building associated with your sleep problem?

Once you have established the root cause of the problem, you can then take the supplements which suit your situation.

If you suffer from hypertension due to worries then a supplement which reduces the hypertension and allows your body to relax and develop a good sleep pattern is essential. Dowse and ask if your sleep pattern would be improved by a supplement of any of the following plant medicine: (1) Black Cohosh, (2)

Chamomile, (3) Hawthorn, (4) Kava Kava, (5) Passion Flower, (6) Valerian, (7) Yarrow, or (8) Vervaine. If you receive a 'Yes' answer then dowse each one separately to find which is the most beneficial supplement. Also dowse and ask if your body is short of Potassium as this mineral helps the body to relax.

The two most common culprits I have found responsible for sleep problems are a shortage of Melatonin and Geopathic Stress. Let's begin by dowsing to ask if you are sleeping over a Geopathic Stress line. If this is confirmed, cleanse your pendulum as ask it to please clear the Geopathic Stress from the building.

Once you have dealt with the Geopathic Stress, it's time to check the Melatonin level in your body. If your pendulum confirms that your body is short of the hormone Melatonin you can ask the pendulum to please top up your body to the correct level with Melatonin as a temporary measure.

Your pineal gland, which is involved in regulating the sleep pattern, produces Melatonin and often when we get elderly our body can become short of this hormone. You cannot purchase this pill in the UK but it is available on the internet and also in the US. I recommend an excellent little book on this subject called *The Melatonin Miracle.*[21] This book was a New York Times bestseller and is crammed full of information about the benefits of this pill, which is non-addictive and guarantees a good night's sleep. The big bonus is that Melatonin boosts the immune system, is an age-reversing, disease fighting and sex enhancing hormone, so it is not surprising that Newsweek say 'It is poised to become one of the hottest pills of the decade'. That's some recommendation!

If your pendulum confirms that your body is short of the hormone Melatonin, ask the pendulum if your pineal gland is working efficiently? If your pineal gland is out of balance you can correct this problem with the pendulum.

Please believe me that in most cases it is possible to improve your sleeping pattern and perhaps one of the above suggestions will resolve your problem.

There are other factors which can also affect your sleep, such as bad Feng Shui in the bedroom or electromagnetic energy from a television or computer. Unless electrical equipment has been unplugged at the wall, it will still give off rays which can disrupt sleep. Another culprit can be a cordless phone which is in the room next to the headboard of your bed, as the base of these phones give off a very powerful energy field.

Dowse and ask if your sleep pattern is disturbed by electromagnetic fields? If the answer is 'Yes', you can dowse each piece of equipment in the room. You can also ask if this negative energy is coming from a nearby telephone mast, overhead power cables or a television satellite.

Does your bedroom have fitted wardrobes with a full length mirror? These create very bad Feng Shui and disrupt sleep. Dowse and ask if the mirrors are disrupting your sleep pattern and if you receive a 'Yes' answer, experiment by hanging a net curtain over the mirror doors at bedtime.

You can also ask if negative energy from outside the building is the culprit. If so, you can purchase a small bagua mirror and hang it outside your building. This little eight sided mirror deflects negative energy which approaches the building.

Negative energy can come from all sorts of sources. Perhaps your home overlooks a busy main road and negative energy is spinning off of traffic as it goes around a roundabout, or accelerates away from traffic lights. The possibilities are endless. If your pendulum confirms that the root cause of your sleep problem is negative energy bombarding your building from an outside factor then it's time to purchase a small bagua mirror. They can be found in most new age shops.

I have given you many avenues to explore and with the aid of your pendulum, you will be able to find the way to a good night's sleep.

IRRITABLE BOWEL SYNDROME

Irritable Bowel Syndrome is a frighteningly common complaint which causes sufferers to experience diarrhoea, constipation, flatulence and tummy pains. This illness causes lots of inconvenience at work and in the social life. It's no exaggeration to say that IBS totally disrupts your everyday life and it can be difficult to control the uncomfortable symptoms.

This illness responds well to meditation, which helps to relax the body and relieves stress. Interestingly, I have found that every person I have treated with this problem suffers from a shortage of chromium. It is worth dowsing to ask if you too are short of this important item. It's usually sold as a small pill and can be purchased from any health shop.

Surprisingly, I have noticed that almost all the sufferers I have treated have shown great and rapid improvement in their symptoms when their home is cleared of Geopathic Stress and they take a supplement of brewers yeast. This inexpensive little pill is crammed full of goodness and can work wonders, so dowse and ask if your health will benefit from taking a supplement of brewers yeast.

Low levels of the Amino Acid Glutathione can be a cause of 'leaky bowel' so dowse and ask if your body is short of Glutathione. Ask if your body would benefit for a supplement of the Amino Acid Glutamine as it can repair the gut lining. Another Amino Acid which is often helpful for this complaint is Cysteine, so ask your pendulum if a supplement of this Amino Acid would be help to reduce symptoms.

The minerals Magnesium, Molybdenum and Selenium can be very important in helping to reduce the symptoms of this complaint, so dowse and ask if a supplement of Molybdenum would help to reduce symptoms and then ask if a supplement of Selenium would benefit your health. Now ask if your body is short of Magnesium? You will probably find that your body does not need supplements of all the above minerals and amino acids, but will certainly benefit from some of them. Your pendulum will guide you as to which are the most beneficial for your body but, as I am not a qualified doctor and only talk from experience of results seen by patients, please check with your doctor before taking any of these supplements.

It is also important to dowse to check that you are not sleeping or working over Geopathic Stress energy, as this is very often linked to irritable bowel syndrome. If you find the presence of this negative energy, you can use the pendulum to clear it by swinging the pendulum and asking it to clear Geopathic Stress from the building and show you the 'Yes' sign when it is clear. The exercise may take five minutes but it will be time well spent – there is an amazing difference in health when this energy has been removed. There will be no more waking up feeling tired and finding your body does not respond to treatment.

Dowse and ask if your Irritable Bowel symptoms are caused by an allergic reaction to certain foods.

1. Are any of my IBS symptoms caused by any foods in my diet?
2. Is my body allergic to Cows milks?
3. Is my body allergic to dairy produce?

If you receive a 'Yes' answer to your symptoms being due to an allergic reaction, but a 'No' answer to milk or dairy food then it's time to make a list of all the foods you eat and drink regularly. You can then dowse each one individually to find the source of the allergy.

Certain dietary supplements can improve IBS symptoms, but each sufferer reacts to different medication depending on their allergies and level of stress. Dowse and ask the following questions:

1. Would a supplement of Lactobacillus (available in health shops) reduce the symptoms?
2. Vitamin B complex is favoured by many sufferers, so ask if your body would benefit from a supplement of vitamin B complex.
3. Would a capsule of peppermint oil reduce symptoms?
4. Ask if the acid/alkaline pH level in your body is balanced?

Many IBS sufferers have an imbalance in this department. In fact, I have found that this is a symptom of most illnesses and when it has been resolved the symptoms reduce rapidly. If your pendulum confirms your body has a pH imbalance, please consider altering your diet to include lots of fruit and green vegetables. These are alkaline and will work to reduce the acid level, which will likely reduce your symptoms.

JOINT PROBLEMS

As we get older, our joints begin to complain and remind us of their existence. There are certain natural treatments which will often successfully remove discomfort. Dowse and ask which of the following supplements will relieve your joint problem. **Chondroitin** is an excellent supplement as a joints and cartilage lubricant.

If the problem is caused by inflamed tissue then **Boswellia** is an invaluable friend. **Glucosamine** is a natural substance found in the cartilage which reduces pain and can often restore mobility. This supplement can be given to animals as well as we humans, and many veterinary surgeons prescribe a pill which contains Glucosamine and other ingredients to our four legged friends who suffer aches and pains.

MSM tablets are a good source of sulphur which repairs tissue, so dowse and ask if your joint pains will be relieved by a supplement of MSM?

If the pain in the joint is linked to scar tissue from an old injury or operation, then I recommend **Serrapeptase,** which removes scar tissue.

KNEES

Painful knees are very debilitating. Every time you change position, they remind you of their presence. There are so many possible causes for pains in knees and dowsing will establish the cause. Perhaps the pain is from an old injury which has flared up, or wear and tear. Other pains can be caused by moving awkwardly and tearing a ligament, an inflamed bursa or arthritis.

Pain can sometimes come from another area, so it's worth checking to ask if the pain is caused by a problem in your spine or pelvis. When my pelvis is out of alignment I often get pains in my knee, which go away as soon as my spine has been manipulated.

If the pain is at the back of the knee then it's possible it could be a problem caused by synovial fluid gathering there, known as Bakers Cyst.

Make a list of all the possibilities and dowse. Here are some suggestions

1. Is the pain caused by Bursitis?
2. Has a ligament in my knee been torn?
3. Has a tendon in my knee been damaged?
4. Is the pain in my knee deferred from my spine?

Dowse and ask if your knee injury would benefit from placing an ice pack on the inflamed area for a few minutes. While heat is more pleasant, chiropractors swear by ice packs, so grit your teeth and you'll soon get used to the cold pack!

Pain in the knee can often be relieved by Chondroitin, Glucosamine, Boswellia or MSM tablets so dowse and ask your pendulum if your knee pain will respond to one of these supplements.

KIDNEY DISEASE

Kidney disease becomes serious when toxic waste collects in the blood and tissues and your kidneys have ceased to act as filters. Many sufferers have no option but to go on a Dialysis machine to clear these problems, but this can often lead to a deficiency of several important minerals, which in itself creates energy and health problems. Kidney disease, particularly kidney failure, may be linked to an imbalance in the level of nickel. Dowse and ask if the level of nickel in your body is wrong? The body only needs a minute amount of nickel but if this is missing it can stop the kidneys running smoothly.

Many sufferers are short of the trace mineral Vanadium, so dowse and ask if your body is deficient in this mineral. Also ask if it is short of the trace mineral Boron.

Ask the pendulum if your body would benefit from a supplement of any of the following: (1) Co Enzyme Q10, (2) Nickel, (3) Vanadium, (4) Manganese, (5) Boron, (6) Melatonin or (7) Vitamin D? Dowse each one separately.

The amino acid L'Carnitine is often lost in dialysis, so it is important to check if your body is short of this important amino acid. The other area to check is the glands as the Pineal gland is often out of balance when kidneys are diseased. Dowse and ask if this gland is out of balance and if so, use the pendulum to create the correct balance.

Many sufferers have for some time been sleeping over Geopathic Stress energy, so dowse and ask if this energy is present in your home or workplace. If you receive a 'Yes' answer then you can use your pendulum to clear the problem.

Have you ever considered that your kidney problem could possibly be linked to something as simple as an acid/alkaline imbalance? When acid waste collects in the blood, it can lead to all sorts of kidney problems and bladder illnesses including Nephritis. It is well worth dowsing to ask if your body's acid/alkaline balance is wrong as this can create problems and stop your body returning to good health. Your pendulum can balance the pH level and, by changing your diet to include fruit and vegetables, you will help to balance this important level. In order to restore the correct pH level with your pendulum, take the following steps.

Ask your pendulum if the acid level in your body is too high? If you receive a 'Yes' answer, you can dowse on a 1–10 scale to find the level of imbalance.

Start by asking if the acid level is above 5 on the 1–10 scale? If the answer is Yes, then ask if it is above 7 on this scale. The correct pH level should always have less acid than alkaline and some experts say your body should be roughly 80% alkaline. There are several very different schools of thought on the right level of pH in the body, so dowse and ask if the correct level of your pH should be below 5? You can dowse and play about with figures until you find the correct level for your good health.

You can then ask your pendulum to please balance the acid/alkaline level in your body and show you the 'Yes' sign when this has been completed.

KIDNEY STONES

It's not surprising that kidney stones can cause breathtaking pain – these stones are made from crystals which have been separated from the urine and form a hard stone.

Kidney stones are not simply a modern day health problem as MedicalNet report scientists have found evidence of kidney stones in a 78,000-year-old Egyptian mummy.[19]

If you suffer severe pain in the urinary system, get out your pendulum and dowse to ask the questions following questions: Is the pain in the urinary tract area caused by a kidney stone? If you receive a 'Yes' answer then you should ask if there is more than one stone present.

When asking about pain location, it is important to always name the area concerned as there could be pain in more than one area in your body, i.e. a stiff neck or a headache, and this could influence the pendulum's answer.

Many sufferers swear by Cranberry juice as it seems to have the natural ability to dissolve the stones in the kidneys. Bearberry juice is also helpful in dissolving them, and sufficient levels of Magnesium in the body can stop stones forming. Dowse and ask your pendulum if Cranberry juice or Bearberry juice will dissolve your stones and also ask if a supplement of Magnesium will stop further stones from forming in your kidneys.

An adequate amount of Potassium, Boron, Vitamins B6 and Vitamin C are helpful, so dowse and ask about your body's levels of each individually.

Devil's Claw Root tea and Nettle tea are also helpful in dealing with this painful problem.

LEG ULCERS

Leg ulcers create very nasty open wounds which can take a long time to heal because they have to heal from the inside. Any assistance from the plant and mineral kingdoms is therefore invaluable.

Ask your pendulum if the sufferer has too high a level of copper in their body? Also ask if they have too high a level of the amino acid Cysteine? If you receive a 'Yes' answer to either of these questions then ask the pendulum to please remove the excess, or ask it to please balance the level and show you the 'Yes' sign when it has finished – this exercise should only take a few minutes.

Bathing the wound with Colloidal silver will help to keep it clear of infection. Dowse and ask if bathing with Colloidal silver will speed up healing?

Gingko Biloba is helpful because it increases the circulation to the leg. Evening Primrose Oil helps to promote improvement while Echinacea strengthens the immune system and enables the body to heal itself faster.

Dowse and ask your pendulum if a supplement of Gingko Biloba, Evening Primrose Oil or Echinacea will help the ulcer to heal? Ask each one separately. Also ask the pendulum if a supplement of Vitamin E capsules, or massaging the body with Vitamin E cream so that it absorbs into the blood will help the ulcers to heal?

When all else fails try the cabbage leaf! This ancient remedy has no side effects and is inexpensive. Remove the hard core from the leaves and place a leaf over the wound. Leave it there overnight to draw the inflammation out of the wound. Cut the toe from an old sock to act as a sleeve to hold the leaf in place. As it is important for the ulcer to heal from the inside outwards, a leaf will be required for many days but you will probably start to notice a difference in the appearance of the wound very quickly.

LIVER PROBLEMS

With many liver problems, it's Rain Forest to the rescue. Devil's Claw Root and Curcuma Root from Java are excellent supplements to purify the liver.

Milk Thistle is truly a friend to all liver sufferers. It has been used in Germany for many years to treat liver complaints and in the treatment of Hepatitis B. Dowse and ask if your liver problems will respond to a supplement of Milk Thistle?

Perhaps there is a problem with the levels of Amino Acids in your body. Please dowse each one of these amino acids and ask if your body is short of any of the following: (1) L'Carnitine, (2) Methionine, (3) Leucine, (4) Cysteine, (5) Isoleuvine or (6) Valine. If the levels of any of this group are low, your pendulum can be used to bring the vibration to the correct level.

Wild Yam, Bearberry juice, Co. Enzyme Q10 and Liquorice are all beneficial to certain liver complaints, so ask if any of these would help to heal the liver. Cirrhosis of the liver occurs when the liver has been scarred by injury or illness and in the case of heavy drinkers, the damage can be due to excess alcohol.

Liver damage caused by Hepatitis C can often be reversed by a combination of Alpha-lipoic acid, Silymarin and Selenium, according to research results at the University of Victoria in Canada.[23]

If anyone in your family suffers from Hepatitis C then dowse and ask if a supplement of Alpha-lipoic acid, Silymarin or Selenium would cure the problem? Also ask the pendulum if this treatment often makes surgery and transplants unnecessary.

The liver is one organ in the body which has the ability to regenerate itself, so it can often recover from serious illness. There are several plants which can support the liver, so dowse and ask the cause of the liver damage and the most effective treatment.

LUPUS

Lupus is an immune system related illness which has unpleasant and restricting symptoms. I have noticed that in many cases the sufferers have a problem with confronting authority. Perhaps they had a difficult relationship with their mother, an over authorative father or a controlling husband or boss. Whoever the cause of this inner rebellion against the authority, it is the illness that causes the body to turn back on itself.

Use your pendulum to check all your chakras are balanced. If any are out of balance then ask the pendulum to balance them.

Check if the Pineal gland is out of balance and if so, use the pendulum to balance this gland.

Some sufferers find Cat's Claw a helpful supplement and others find Melatonin is useful, so dowse and ask if either of these supplements will improve your symptoms. Certain Lupus sufferers have used the enzyme from the venom of the Russell's Pit Viper, so ask if a supplement of this venom would improve the symptoms of the illness. If you receive a 'Yes' sign, ask the pendulum to channel the correct amount to you. It may sound awful, but then so is the illness – if it is going to help to reduce the symptoms then try not to think that it is from a snake!

MALARIA

Malaria is a disease which claims millions of lives each year and ruins the holiday of many travellers. Is there any cure for this illness?

The answer seems to be Yes, in the form of the Wormwood plant, an effective weapon against Malaria. This little known plant contains Artemisinin, which has been proved in clinical trials in China to be 90% effective – more effective than standard drugs.[16]

In a trial involving 2,000 patients, all of those suffering from Malaria were cured by this plant. If you ever suffer from Malaria, remember the Wormwood plant![37]

Further confirmation that the Wormwood is bad news for Malaria is a report that extracts from the Chinese herb Quinghoa, or Sweet Wormwood (Artemisia Annua), has the ability to disable the parasite.[20] It is available from Chinese Herbalists. Dowse and ask:

1. Will a supplement of Wormwood reduce my symptoms of Malaria?
2. Will a supplement of Wormwood clear my symptoms of Malaria?
3. Can a supplement of the Brazilian Cinchona Bark reduce symptoms?

It is useful to know a treatment for Malaria before you are ever infected, so if your pendulum confirms Wormwood or Cinchona are beneficial, it may be worth enquiring if Wormwood medication can be taken on your travels.

Cinchona is a natural cure for Malaria used by the local people. It is also known as Peruvian Bark, which is found in the Amazon. This tree gives us quinine from its bark.

ME – Myalgic Encephalomyelitis/CFS – Chronic Fatigue Syndrome

This post viral fatigue syndrome is at last being recognised as a genuine illness after many years of being referred to as the Yuppie Flu. It is difficult for doctors to diagnose this illness as symptoms vary, but the one thing sufferers have in common is a feeling of incredible exhaustion. Sometimes they don't even have the energy to get out of bed. Other symptoms include a red blood flow in parts of the chain which changes chemistry.

When I treat a person who suffers from ME, I start by clearing their home of Geopathic Stress from underground water. The rays from the water are usually present where ME sufferers sleep.

Once I have removed any negative energy from the home I then balance the Ions and then the pineal gland, as this gland is often out of balance. You can dowse to ask for then presence of Geopathic Stress and also to ask your pendulum if the pineal gland is out of balance.

I then check the body for any deficiencies of minerals. This is a task you can do with a friend. Start by checking if your body has excess nickel? Also ask the pendulum if your body has excess histamine? If you receive a 'Yes' answer to either question, ask the pendulum to please balance the level of nickel or histamine. All balancing can be done very effectively with the pendulum as long as both your energy and the pendulum's energy are free of negativity.

Beetroot is very beneficial as it helps to build blood. Echinacea will help to rebuild the immune system. The following also play an important part in fighting ME. Dowse each of the following separately to ask if your body would benefit from a supplement of:

(1) Potassium, (2) Magnesium, (3) Echinacea, (4) Iodine, (5) Melatonin, (6) Aloe Vera, (7) Co Enzyne Q10, and (8) L'Carnitine.

As everybody needs slightly different medication, dowse and ask each of the following questions.

1. Ask the pendulum if there is Geopathic Stress in your home.
2. Ask the pendulum if beetroot will improve your body's blood supply.
3. Will Echinacea help your body to fight ME?
4. Can Ginkgo Biloba help reduce ME symptoms?
5. Will a course of Melatonin improve ME symptoms? (*Available on the web.*)
6. Can Aloe Vera improve my symptoms?
7. Is my body short of magnesium?
8. Is my pineal gland out of balance?
9. Is the Acid/Alkaline level in my body balanced?
10. Does my body have excess nickel?
11. Does my body have excess histamine?
12. Can a supplement of Evening Primrose reduce symptoms?

You will find that you get positive answers to some of the questions. You should then get a friend or relative to dowse to confirm the answers.

Some ME sufferers will find that it's Propolis to the rescue! In a trial involving 27 chronically ill patients who all suffered from ME some had shown great response after taking a supplement of Propolis for one week. After four months of taking this supplement, 24 of these patients had received major benefit.[28] Dowse and ask if a supplement of Propolis would reduce your ME symptoms?

Some sufferers of ME have such a weak immune system that they can acquire a negative attachment which takes their energy. This happens when the aura has a gap or crack, enabling the entity to move in. Ask someone to dowse to ask if you have any form of negative attachment. The big problem is that if you have an attachment stealing your energy, you will not get correct dowsing answers. To be on the safe side, ask a friend to check this important question.

Many ME sufferers have found that Propolis gives great improvement to symptoms, so dowse and ask if this natural substance would reduce your symptoms? Propolis is a substance which comes from tree bark and has been used for many centuries to fight a range of illnesses. It is beneficial to Arthritis, Acne, Blood Pressure problems, Bronchitis, Candida Albican, gastro intestinal problems and many other illnesses.

Are you concerned that perhaps your heart is not functioning correctly, which could account for the overwhelming tiredness? Dowse and ask if your heart is functioning properly and then ask if it's in good working order.

Dr Arnold Peckerman's research showed that when standing upright, the blood of ME sufferers is pumping one and a half litres per minute slower than a healthy person's heart and when lying down, their blood is pumping two litres per minute slower than the heart of a healthy person, which certainly accounts for the feeling of weakness.[25] Cleanse your pendulum and then dowse and ask if the weakness symptom of your body is linked to mitochondrial malfunction? If you receive a 'Yes' answer, you can ask your pendulum to please balance the level of mitochondrial and show you the 'Yes' sign when completed.

Another consideration is the presence of environmental toxins, including heavy metals, pesticides and air pollutants in the body. Dowse and ask if your body has a harmful level of any toxic heavy metals including mercury, arsenic, or lead. Then ask the same questions for pesticides, chemicals and air pollutants as many sufferers of ME blame the presence of these unwelcome nuisances.

Many of us think of ME as an adult illness but sadly there are an enormous number of children who suffer from this debilitating illness and miss long periods of school. In the UK alone the Department of Health figures show that 25,000 children suffer from ME, and at least 50% of long term absences from school are due to ME.

Contact 'Action for ME' if you would like further information on this illness. Email: wells@afme.org.uk[31]

MENOPAUSE PROBLEMS

Some women are fortunate enough to sail through the menopause virtually free of unpleasant symptoms, while others experience several years of suffering all sorts of uncomfortable symptoms. So is there any natural cure for this unseen ailment that gets little sympathy and is often a music hall joke?

The first things to check are the Pituitary gland and the Hypothalmus gland. One or both of these glands are often out of balance in sufferers, so ask your pendulum the question 'is my Pituitary gland out of balance?' Now repeat the question for the Hypothalamus gland, and if the answer is 'Yes' for either then use the pendulum to balance the gland and ask to be shown the 'Yes' sign when it has been done.

Many women find relief from symptoms with a supplement of the herbal remedy Black Cohosh, which is thought to regulate the

Lutenising hormone. Boron is also a helpful supplement as it helps calcium intake, which is important to the body at this time. Dowse and ask if your menopausal symptoms would be reduced by a supplement of Black Cohosh? Would your body benefit from extra Boron?

Premenstrual tension

Premenstrual tension can be a living nightmare to some women and the families who are at the receiving end of their tension. Agnus Castus is the answer, along with B complex which helps to control tension.

Some problems can be caused by excess estrogen and a deficiency of progesterone, so ask your pendulum if this is the problem. If so, ask it to balance them.

Is your body short of Essential Fatty acids? A shortage of Zinc or Magnesium can also cause tension. Would you benefit from extra Boron? Dowse for answers.

It is amazing how taking a supplement of Magnesium can control mood changes. Other minerals also play a big part in reducing the symptoms.

Dowse and find out which supplements will reduce the tension, as there is no point in suffering in silence! Irregular periods often occur as a symptom of the menopause, or if you are run down. This upset of the cycle can be helped by one of the following plants: Agnus Castus, Dong Qui or Ginseng. Dowse and ask if your cycle would be helped by one or more of these plants?

MIGRAINE

Any migraine sufferer will tell you this is a nightmare period as their life stands still. When the migraine strikes them, they are often housebound for several days and feeling very antisocial. They all describe an awful feeling of nausea and sensitivity to light, with some reporting a bright aura around objects. So what is the cause of migraines?

The causes are many and varied and can be brought on by a hormone disruption, a neck or cranial injury or sleeping over a Geopathic Stress line. If you suffer from migraines then dowse and ask if the migraine is instigated by a hormone imbalance? If you receive a 'Yes' answer, you can then ask if the level of progesterone is too high, and depending on the answer you can ask if it is too low. Dowse to check if the estrogen level is wrong. Try your question a few times and when you are confident the answer is correct, you can ask the pendulum to please balance the hormone level and show you the 'Yes' sign when the job is complete.

Next, ask your pendulum if you are sleeping or working over Geopathic Stress. If a 'Yes' answer you can ask if the migraine is linked to the Geopathic Stress energy?

If this negative energy is present, it is a simple job for your pendulum to clear this energy from your home or workplace.

What medication can you take to avoid having a migraine? And what treatments can reduce this painful experience? Feverfew is an excellent friend to sufferers as it prevents the migraine becoming established. Vitamin B2 Riboflavin reduces the severity of the attack and many sufferers find that taking Vitamin B12 each morning can stop them. Migraine sufferers are very often short of Magnesium, so dowse and ask if your body has a magnesium deficiency?

MSM sulphur tablets are a good supplement for sufferers and Damiana is also helpful. Guarana helps the body to relax and feel good so is a useful pill to have in the cupboard. Dowse and ask: would Damiana or Guarana help your body to recover from a migraine? Would cranial osteopathy reduce the number of attacks? Then ask your pendulum: is the problem caused by a neck injury? If the answer is 'Yes' then ask if a chiropractor would be able to release the pressure which is causing the problem.

A Migraine is a painful experience but perhaps some of the above suggestions will help to reduce your discomfort.

Headaches

Today, headaches are a frighteningly common complaint and many are caused by the stress of modern day living. The World Health Organisation report that roughly two thirds of men and 80% of women suffer from regular headaches and one in every 20 adults suffer a headache almost every day.[24]

When you feel the first sign of a dreaded headache approaching it's often an automatic reaction to reach for the painkillers but if you regularly suffer from headaches, it is well worth taking evasive action to prevent this nuisance. Headaches can often be prevented by a supplement of B vitamins as they reduce stress, thereby reducing headaches. Another vitamin which is a good friend to headache sufferers is vitamin E, which increases circulation and helps strengthen the immune system.

Cinchona (Peruvian Bark) can be a useful supplement, while Valerian Root or Feverfew will improve your quality of sleep. Feverfew is also helpful is reducing the number of migraine headaches you suffer.

Headaches can be caused by an allergic reaction to certain foods, to stress at work, family tension, etc., but one cause which is seldom mentioned is sleeping over Geopathic Stress. Many sufferers have found that when this energy has been cleared from their home or workplace, they no longer suffer from headaches and awaken feeling fit and fresh each morning. Dowse the following questions:

1. Am I sleeping or working over Geopathic Stress energy? If you receive a 'Yes' answer, ask your pendulum to clear this energy.
2. Ask if your headache is caused by an Acid/Alkaline imbalance?
3. If your headache is caused by a digestive problem, ask the pendulum if Acidophilus would reduce the problem?
4. Dowse and ask if your body would benefit from a supplement of any of the following supplements:

(1) Magnesium, (2) Chromium, (3) Cinchona, (4) Vitamin E, (5) Vitamin B's, (6) Kava Kava, (7) Potassium, (8) Zinc, (9) Copper or (10) Calcium. Dowse each one separately.

There are so many possible causes of headaches, so dowse and find the cause, along with the most helpful treatment for headaches, and stop them disrupting your life.

MULTIPLE CHEMICAL SENSITIVITY

It's generally accepted by scientists that multiple chemical sensitivity is on the increase and, according to noted NASA scientist Dr B.C. Wolverton, figures are expected to increase by 60% before 2010. The Institute of Medicine have estimated that one in five folks in North America will experience an allergen type illness during their lifetime and 28% of Americans experience Multiple Chemical Sensitivity (MSC).[26] The atmosphere, both indoors and outdoors, is like a sea of pollution and there seem to be very few methods of reducing this pollution. The pollution can come from a wide range of sources including industry, furnishings and household cleaning products.

So what can we do to reduce pollution in our homes? The first good rule is to try and avoid all perfume products and the second rule is to place plants in your home and office. Plants have a natural ability to absorb pollution, particularly Spider plants which are very easy to care for. They are a must in rooms where electromagnetic fields are present from computers and electronic equipment. Plants are the lungs of our earth – they produce oxygen, which we need to survive.

MULTIPLE SCLEROSIS

Multiple Sclerosis (MS) is an autoimmune disease which affects the brain and the spinal cord of the sufferer. When the central nervous system is damaged, it can then trigger a range of unpleasant symptoms; the body's immune system, instead of fighting infections, attacks the myelin sheath and leads to a serious breakdown in messages. It is by far the most common neurological disease suffered by young people and the Multiple Sclerosis Society confirm there are 85,000 sufferers in the UK alone.

MS sufferers often have a low level of Histamine in their body, so dowse and check if the levels of Histamine need to be balanced. Also ask your pendulum if your body would benefit from extra Phospherous, as this is helpful in fighting muscle fatigue. Potassium is another useful mineral to fight muscle fatigue, which is why you often see tennis players at Wimbledon eating bananas on the court. Ask the pendulum if a supplement of potassium would improve muscle fatigue? Many MS sufferers are deficient in Vitamin B12, so ask if your body would benefit from a supplement of this vitamin.

The mineral Molybdenum helps some sufferers and Cat's Claw is often found to reduce symptoms, so dowse and ask if either of them would help to reduce the MS symptoms.

Studies at Oxford University have shown Propolis as a useful treatment of MS and other autoimmune illnesses and there are no side effects. Dowse and ask if a supplement of Propolis would reduce some MS symptoms?[27]

There is a school of thought which says that a number of MS cases are caused by a malfunction in the myelin sheath caused by the measles virus.

Dowse and ask if damage done by this virus is linked to MS? If you receive a 'Yes' answer then ask the pendulum to please remove the vibration of this virus from the body. If you doubt this is possible, then ask the pendulum if it is able to do this task.

It is always worth asking your pendulum to check the level of heavy metals in your body, particularly mercury. If an excess is present then ask the pendulum to please remove the excess.

MS in males

Will extra testosterone help to reduce symptoms in men suffering relapsing remitting symptoms of MS? Research carried out at the University of California Los Angeles (UCLA) showed that symptoms improved when testosterone gel was applied to the arm each day. More research in this treatment is needed, but results so far are promising. Dowse and ask if any male sufferer in your family would benefit from the application of testosterone gel on their arm?[18]

MUSCULAR/BONE AND JOINT PROBLEMS

Most of us suffer sprains, lacerations, bone spurs and bone fractures at some time in our life, so it is helpful to know of alternative remedies which help to speed up healing of these problems. They all require different medication, so here are a few natural treatments which folks find beneficial.

A **sprain** is a very painful injury and can be relieved with Arnica cream and pills, Alfalfa or Comfrey. St John's Wort helps to relax the injured area and speed up healing, while a cabbage leaf placed over the wound overnight draws out inflammation. Keeping it in place can be difficult so I always cut the toe off an old sock and pull it over the limb to keep the leaf in place. Dowse and ask if the injury would respond to Alfalfa. Then ask if it would also benefit from Comfrey.

Bone Spurs are very inconvenient as they usually appear on the heel and make walking painful. Some therapists say they are caused by a Calcium imbalance, so dowse and ask if the level of calcium in your body is too low? Or too high? If you receive a 'Yes' answer, ask the pendulum to please balance the calcium level in your body and show you the 'Yes' sign when it has been completed.

Lacerations – wounds. Nettle Tea is excellent for slowing the bleeding in a wound. Cleanse with Witch Hazel, Echinacea, Tea Tree lotion or Colloidal Silver solution. When the wound occurs outdoors you can use a Yarrow leaf or Dock Leaf to stop the bleeding. These plants are to be found in most green areas and are part of nature's 'first aid' kit. Dowse and ask if Yarrow or Dock Leaf will stem the bleeding?

Bone Fractures are an injury which merits a visit to the casualty department at your local hospital, but before you get there you can use Arnica to reduce the bruising. Alfalfa and Comfrey help to heal bone fractures, so dowse and ask if your injury would benefit from a supplement of these gentle treatments which have no side effects.

Boswellia can reduce inflamed tissue and Chondroitin is very helpful for lubricating joints and cartilage, while Glucosamine helps to rebuild cartilage and restore fluidity. Dowse and ask if any of the above will benefit your injury or ache?

Today there's a great selection of treatments available for muscle and joint aches, but there's a lot to be said for using old fashioned treatments. I can well remember my grandmother using Epsom Salts in the bath to relieve aches and I have many times followed her example and soaked in a bath containing Epsom Salts to relieve a backache.

So how does the Epsom Salt treatment work? It's all about balancing the acid/alkaline level. The Epsom Salts soak through the skin into the bloodstream.

Folks whose body is more acid than alkaline can create balance by adding a cup of Epsom Salts and 2 pints of Apple Cider Vinegar into their bath water. This will soak through the skin and improve the Acid/Alkaline balance. Many arthritis sufferers swear by Apple Cider Vinegar, so dowse and ask if this treatment will relieve your aches.

Dowse and ask if your body's Acid/Alkaline level is out of balance? If your body has a high level of Acid then, by adjusting your diet, you can create a more permanent balance.

NANO TECHNOLOGY AND HEALTH

Look Out! Nanotechnology is about! Most of us are only vaguely aware of nanotechnology and few of us could describe this new science which is rapidly placing genetic engineering in the shade. The ETC Group describe nanotechnology as referring to a spectrum of new technologies involving the manipulation of matter at the scale of atoms and molecules. A nanometre is one billionth of a metre so we are talking about an almost invisible technology.

Nanotechnology has instigated an intensifying race to file nano tech patent applications so governments need to urgently evaluate the impact of this new science on human health. Warning! There are no regulations explicitly targeting nanotechnology anywhere in the world. Yes the subject is being discussed, but already hundreds of nano-products are available with countless others in the pipeline, all with no regulations! We must ask the question '*Is science opening a Pandora's Box of unforeseen and uncontrollable consequences?*' Have the world's governments listened to the warning from Swiss Re, the world's second largest re insurance bank, who've warned of unknown and unpredictable risks which could make nanotechnology uninsurable?[33]

Is nanotechnology affecting our health? Is this new science of nano-particles a force to be reckoned with? The latest toxic warning has shown that nano-particles cause brain damage in aquatic species, which certainly highlights the urgent need for a moratorium on the release of nano-materials. A report commissioned by the European Parliament states that nano-particles should not be released into the environment as recent studies have raised concern about the toxicity of these particles.

At the American Chemical Society's National Meeting, Dr Eva Oberdorster described an experiment when she exposed nine largemouth bass in water containing buckyballs (carbon molecules). After 48 hours, the fish were found to have suffered severe brain damage in the form of lipid peroxidation. This is a condition which leads to destruction of cell membranes similar to Alzheimer's disease.[32(a)]

Dowse and ask the following questions:

1. Can any particular nano-particles damage human health?
2. Can any nano-particles cause brain damage in humans?
3. Will nanotechnology cause an increase in illnesses?
4. Will any nano-particles affect our glands?

5. Can buckyballs (*carbon molecules*) cross the blood brain barrier?
6. Will buckyballs eventually get into our food chain?
7. Are buckyballs already ingredients in food on sale in food stores?
8. Can buckyballs soak through our skin into our blood?

There's plenty of work for your pendulum as nano-particles measuring a few billionths of a metre are already in commercial products on sale, including anti-aging cream, sunblocks, car body parts and tennis rackets. Dr Oberdorster warns '*We are already aware that buckyballs can cross the blood brain barrier in humans*', so are scientists playing with a time bomb? She also reports that these buckyballs are toxic to water fleas; in a test, half of the water fleas died within 2 days. This is not a good sign as water fleas are a food source for other aquatic species. Could this be the start of buckyballs in our food chain?

Research has shown that nano-particles can easily move from nasal passageways to the brain[32(b)] and another study showed that these particles can easily be absorbed by earthworms[32(c)], so it is not too difficult to believe they can get into the food chain and into humans.

Confirmation that we are quite right to be apprehensive about nanotechnology comes from the German Federal Institute of Risk, who report magic nano on aerosol, household glass and ceramic cleaner has been recalled after receiving reports of 97 incidents in which this nano product was linked to respiratory disorders.

Dowsing will confirm if a product contains nano ingredients, so until such a time as labelling ingredients becomes compulsory, dowsing is the only way to locate the presence of nano materials.[43]

1. Dowse and ask if the product contains any nano particles.
2. Does it contain more than one group of nano particles?
3. Does the product contain any harmful ingredients?

If you receive a 'Yes' sign, you can cleanse your pendulum and ask it to please remove the vibration of the nano ingredient. The fact that Swiss Re state this new technology is not a good insurance risk does suggest it should be avoided when possible.

The market for nanotechnology is already over one billion dollars which is alarming, for as yet neither regulations nor labelling requirements exist in any country.

In Japan, scientists are experimenting with using buckyballs for agricultural fertiliser.[32] This is not good news as runoff is already polluting many waterways. Could buckyballs run into water supplies? Get dowsing on nanotechnology. It's better to know the danger and be safe rather than sorry!

Already there is great public concern and over millions of websites on this subject. It's time to call governments in all 6 continents to take action. Concern for human safety, and particularly those two million who are expected to work in this industry by 2015, has instigated action from concerned organisations. On July 31st 2007 a Consortium of over forty groups, consumer groups, public health and civil societies from around the world have formed a Coalition and released the Principles for the oversight of Nanotechnologies and Nanomaterials from six continents. All that is needed now is for governments to set these guidelines in motion and to ensure that they are carried out! Here are the details of the much needed guidelines:

1. Manufacturers and distributors must give proof of safety in their product.
2. There must be prevention of exposure to nanoproducts that have not been proven safe, to protect the public and workers.
3. A full lifecycle analysis of environmental impact must be completed prior to commercialisation.
4. All new products must be labelled and nano-industries must be accountable for liabilities incurred from their products.[41]

It's good news for all of us that some regulations may be introduced, but will they be effective? Dowse and ask if these suggestions will be instigated and also ask your pendulum if this technology will be policed by an international body, to ensure we are all protected from unknown dangers. Most of us are confused about the work of 'new science' so here are brief descriptions.

1. Biotechnology is the name of the science which contributes to life by the manipulation of genes, i.e. Dolly the sheep.
2. Nanotechnology is the science used to control matter by manipulating atoms.
3. Cognitive Neuroscience is the name given to the technique of manipulating neurons.

In other words, these new sciences have all overtaken genetic engineering. We are going to hear a lot more about then within the next few years.

DOUBTFUL TECHNOLOGY!

Building Life Form from Scratch?

We think Nanotechnology is advanced science, but synthetic biology leaves it well behind! Can synthetic life cause long term damage to civilisation?

Synthetic biology is a controversial new field of science. You must admit, it is rather ambitious to attempt to put together the first entirely human made organism. It's not really surprising that international societies and groups are demanding rapid control of this new biology; it sounds as though they are in distinct competition with God!

Building life form from scratch does not sound like a good idea to me – I wonder if the scientists involved have ever considered the long term effect of an army of these DIY life forms? We've all seen science fiction movies with strange looking robots but we don't ever expect that it could become real. However, the possibilities are endless for this new science. Perhaps the most alarming fact is that no laws have yet been developed that address the social safety or security risks.

This new technology, as with nanotechnology, is storming ahead quietly with no governments or international body able to regulate or control it reports Biologist Florianne Koechcia of the Swiss Working Group on Gene Technology.

There is an urgency to lay down rules and guidelines on this biology. A patent application has already been filed on a 'fully synthetic life form' produced via synthetic biology. This patent claims monopoly ownership of a free, living organism that can grow and replicate.

The owner of this trillion dollar patent is proudly reporting that when this project is complete in a few weeks time, it will mark a break with evolution as we know it. But do any of us really want a break with evolution? Such a patent raises the question 'Could it be used in the future by bio-terrorists in germ warfare?'[42] Already there is great public concern and over millions of websites on this subject calling all governments in 6 continents to take action.

References

1. 'Causes of Low Sperm Count' *Baby Hopes*.
   http://www.babyhopes.com
2. 'Erectile Problems and Cycling Under Spotlight'. Aug. 25th 2005.
   http://www.altpenis.com
3. *Rachel's Democracy & Health News* No. 514. 'Chemicals Linked to Declining Male Reproductive Health'. Oct. 96. Peter Montague, (National Writers Union. UAW Local/1981/AFL-C10.
   Ibid – Jorma Toppari & others. 'Male Reproductive Health and Environmental Xenoestrogens. *Environmental Health Perspectives*. Vol. 104. Supplement 741–803. This new report is a revised and abridged version of a report originally commissioned by the Danish Environmental Protection Agency. Copenhagen (*See REHW #438*).
   Ibid – Ted Schettler, Gina Solomon, Paul Burns & Maria Valenti, 'Generations at Risk, How Environmental Toxins May Affect Reproductive Health in Massachusetts.' Greater Boston Physicians for Social Responsibility. www.rachel.org
4. *Rachel's Environment & Health News #752*. The Latest Hormone Science'. Part 3, Sept 19th 2002. 1997/98. NZ Total Diet Survey, Ministry of Health. 'Pesticides Found in Food Linked to Birth Defects'.

5. *Environmental Health Perspectives*, Vol. 103: 582–587. 'Environmental Causes of Infertility' Richard W. Pressinger. M. Ed., Wayne Sinclair M.D. (Board Certified Immunology over past 40 years).
   Ibid – Dr Cecil Jacobson. Reproductive Genetic Center, Virginia.
   Ibid – Dr Pat McShane Dept.of Obstetrics & Gynaecology, Boston Massachusetts '40% of all Infertility Cases Due to the Male'.
   Ibid – Dr Samuel S. Epstein, David Ozonoff. School of Public Health, University of Illinois Medical Center Boston University School of Public Health 'Most Families Live in Pesticide Contaminated Homes' *Teratogenesis, carcinogenesis & Mutagenesis* Vol. 7: 5–7–540.
   Ibid – Dr Eli Gea, 'In Vitro Fertilization Unit, Serlin Maternity Hospital, Tel Aviv. *Fertility Sterility Journal* 62 (4).
   Ibid – Time Magazine Oct. 22 1992 page 27.
   Ibid – Dr Salim Daya, The Fertility Clinic, Chedoke-McMaster Hospital, Ontario. *Chatelaine Magazine.* Nov. 93.
   Ibid – Drs Susan Jobling, Tracey Reynolds, Roger White, Malcolm Parker and John Sumpter. Dept of Biology & Biochemistry, Laboratory of the Molecular Endocrinology, Brunel University, London.
6. 'Pesticides Mimic Human Hormones, Damage Reproductive Systems' 'Environmental Causes of Infertility'. Richard W. Pressinger M.Ed. Wayne Sinclair MD.
   Ibid – Dr Richard M. Sharpe of University of Edinburgh, and Dr Neils Skakikebaek, University of Copenhagen.
   Ibid Dr John A. McLachlan, Director, Intramural Search, Nat. Institute of Environmental Health Services.
7. 'Pesticides Causing Infertility in the Heartland, Country Living may be Hazardous to Men's Fertility' by Orna Izakson. *The Environmental Magazine.* Epidemiologist Shanna Swan. Organic Consumers Association. April 2nd 2004.
   http://www.organicconsumers.org/foodsafety/fertility040504.cfm
8. 'Infertility Linked to Pesticide Exposure' E. Tielemans., R. Van Kooij., E.R. te Velde., A. Burdorf., D. Heederik. 'Pesticide Exposure and Decreased Fertilization Rates in Vitro' *The Lancet.* Vol. 254. 484–85. Positive News No. 45. The Pesticide Trust now Pan UK. http://pan-uk.org
9. 'Disposable Nappies Behind Increase in Male Infertility' Study *The Archives of Disease in Children.* 2000:83:364
   http://www.altpenis.com *The Pharmaceutical Journal.* Vol. 265. No. 7120 Male Infertility Linked with Disposable Nappies.
   http://www.pjonlinbe.com
10. 'Infertility affects 2.5 million males in the UK' Norwich Union Healthcare. *Medical News Today.* Christina Nordquist, Editor.
   http://www.medicalnewstoday.com 13th Sept 2005.

11. 'Avoiding Soya May Aid Fertility' June 21st 2005. Michelle Roberts. *BBC News, World Edition. BBC News Health reporter in Copenhagen.* http://news.bbc.co.uk/2/hi/health/4115506.stm

12. 'Pesticides Linked to Male Infertility' *BBC News.* http://news.bbd.co.uk/l/hi/health/1458660.stm

13. *The Daily Mail Archives.* Beyond Pesticides, 'Study Links Herbicide Use to Infertility in Women'. http://www.beyondpesticides.org

14. *The Collaborative on Health and the Environment.* A.R. Greenlee., T.E. Arbuckle and P.H. Chyou. 'Risk Factor for Female Infertility in an Agricultural Region' *Epidemiology* 14:429–436.

15. 'Semen Quality Affected by Exposure to Pesticides' Beyond Pesticides. http://www.beyondpesticides.org

16. Wormwood. Regenerative Nutrition, 1 The Avenue House Developments, Sark, Channel Islands GY9 OSB UK. Tel 0845 034 5139. http://www.regenerativenutrition.com

17. Dr Joseph Mercola. 'Scientists Warn – Dangerous Chemicals Found in Plastic' www.mercola.com Seattle Times. Aug. 3, 2007. Reproductive Toxicology August 3, 2007.

18. MedicineNet.com 'Testosterone May Help Treat MS in Men'.

19. MedicineNet.com 'Kidney Stones in Adults'. http://www.medicinenet.com

20. Nexus New Times Vol. 10. No. 6. New Scientist Vol. 179 issue 2409. 23rd Aug 2003. Global News.

21. The Melatonin Miracle. Pocket Books. By William Pierpaoli, M.D. Ph.D., and William Regelson M.D. with Carol Colman.

22. Greater Boston Physicians for Social Responsibility with a grant from Jessie B. Cox Charitable Trust. Physician Fact Sheet Reproductive Health & Environment Exposure (619) 497–7440 GBPSR.

23. Nexus New Times. Vol. 11. No. 1. 'Aids The Seleno Enzyme Solution. Harold D. Foster. PhD Professor Dept. of Geography, University of Victoria BC Canada.

24. The World Health Organization. 'How Common are Headaches'. Sept. 30th 2005. Online Q & A.

25. Green Health Watch Magazine. www.greenhealthwatch.com 'ME CFS –Let Down by Faulty Batteries' (12467) Dr Sarah Myhill.

26. Second Hand Radiation, 'Plants Help Reverse Indoor Air Pollution and Allergies. Kootenai Valley Times – Oct. 2000. Dr Gloria Gilbere. www.ourlittleplace.com

27. Regenerative Nutrition http://www.regenerativenutrition.com Penny Hill, July 1987. Sunday Express.

28. Regenerative Nutrition http://www.regenerativenutrition.com Dr J.M. Grange. 'Propolis'.

29. American Autoimmune Related Diseases Association. 'NIH Awards $51 Million to Fight Autoimmune Diseases'. http://www.aarda.org
30. American Autoimmune Related Diseases Association. 'New Study Linking Asbestos to Autoimmunity is Preliminary, But Promising Says American Autoimmune Related Disease Association. http://www.aarda.org
31. Nicole Martin Daily Teleggraph 12.1.02. Independent Weekly Review 16.1.02(8924). http://www.ehn.clara.net/illnesses. html Green Health Watch 'Illness of our time'.
32. Organic Consumers Association. 'Nano Particles Shown to Cause Brain Damage' Genotype, 1st April 2004. www.etcgroup.org
http://www.organicconsumers.org
(a) Mark. T. Sampson 'Type of Buckyball Shown to Cause Brain Damage in Fish' Eurekalert. March 21st 2004. www.eurekalert.org
(b) Geoff Brumfiel 'A Little Knowledge' Nature. Vol. 424. No. 6946, Page 246 July 2003.
(c) Alex Kirby 'Tiny Particles Threaten Brain' BBC News Online. http://www.bbc.co.uk/1/hi/sci/tech/3379759.stm
33. ETC Group '26 Governments Tiptoe Towards Global Nano Governance' Grey Governance. 30th June 2004. www.etcgroup.org
34. What the Doctors Don't Tell You, WDDTY. Oct. 98. Vol. 9, No. 7.
35. What the Doctors Don't Tell You, WDDTY. June 98. Vol. 9, No. 3.
36. Dental Amalgam Fillings Page. Bernie Windham, Editor. http://www.home.earthlink.net
37. Regenerative Nutrition, Wormwood (Artemisia Absinthium). http://www.regnerativenutrition.com
38. JAMA 284 (4) July 2000.
39. Environment and Health News. Vol. 3. June 98. the Ecologist Campaigns & News. April 98.
40. Dr Joseph Mercola. 'What Are These Drugs Doing to You?'. www.mercola.com
41. The ETC Group. 'Broad International Coalition Issues Urgent Call for Strong Oversight of Nanotechnology'. July 31st 2007. http://www.etcgroup.org
42. The Genomes of Zurich: Civil Society Calls for Urgent Controls of Synthetic Life. June 25th 2007. http://www.etcgroup.org
43. Courtesy of Alternative Medicine. No. No, Magic Nano by James Keough. Sept. 2006. http://www.alternativemedicine.com

OBESITY

Obesity is becoming more common every year and, although there is constant publicity in magazines and newspapers on the health effects of this problem, those who suffer seriously still find it difficult to lose weight. So what is wrong with their bodies?

In a few cases, the problem can be caused by a virus which has taken up residence – dowse and ask if the A-D-36 virus is present in your body. If it is present, ask your pendulum to please remove it.

Some sufferers have a defective sebaceous gland, so dowse and ask if your sebaceous gland is functioning correctly and is balanced. If the pendulum confirms this gland is experiencing problems, then ask the pendulum to please balance this gland.

Perhaps the level of the hormone Leptin is wrong? Ask the pendulum to please check if the level of this important hormone is balanced and if not, to please correct the balance. Certain obese people are depleted in the Amino Acid Methionine, so ask if the level is wrong, and if so, it's a job for the pendulum!

Obese people often complain of an uncontrollable urge to eat sweet biscuits and cakes, or an urge to eat chocolate. These are sure signs that the body is short of Chromium. If you find yourself searching every cupboard in an effort to find sweet biscuits or going to a local shop late at night to get a chocolate supply, it is usually a sign that your body is short of B12.

If you experience these cravings for cakes and biscuits, dowse and ask if your symptoms will be reduced by taking Chromium pills for a few days. There is a strong possibility you will be amazed by how quickly the craving vanishes. You only need to take them again for a few days when you feel the first warning signs. I always keep Chromium tablets in the house and take them when I get cravings.

Chocolate craving is often linked to a shortage of B Vitamins, so B12 or B Complex will most likely solve the problem. Before taking a supplement of Chromium or B Vitamins, dowse and ask your pendulum if your body is short of them?

Ask the health shop about Lycopodium by Nelson's. This helps curb the desire for sweet things. Another option is that your body is short of the Amino Acid L'Glutamine, so ask your pendulum if your body is low in this item and ask it to top up to the correct level. There are many causes of obesity. In some folks it may be a case of living on a diet of fattening food, but for those with cravings, hopefully you will have found help here.

OSTEOARTHRITIS

Osteoarthritis affects many people in middle age and is linked to wear and tear of the joints. The symptoms vary from backache to aches in other joints, due to deterioration of cartilage.

I was horrified when a blind physiotherapist I visited for backache told me I had osteoarthritis but, in the next breath, he told me it was nothing to worry about as exercise would hold it all together! He explained that most folks over 40 years of age develop this problem, as the back of ancient man was only designed to last till that age.

Alfalfa is a great treatment for this painful problem and I have met many folks who swear by this grass, which can be purchased in tablet form. Cattle and rabbits love it – they know what's good for their health.

I take supplements of Boswellia, which has powerful anti inflammatory effect, and Chondroiton sulphate. They are both wonderfully effective for improving problems of the joints and ligaments.

A daily supplement of Cat's Claw can attack the problem. This truly amazing anti-inflammatory plant can heal a large number of complaints. Many sufferers take MSM sulphur, which is well known for successfully relieving pain and cleansing the blood. Like the others I have mentioned it is usually free from side effects.

Glucosamine sulphate is probably the best known treatment for muscles and is even used in veterinary pills. You will not require to take all of the supplements I have mentioned so your pendulum will guide you to the most beneficial supplement for your particular ache.

Dowse each supplement separately, asking if it would improve your symptoms of Osteoarthritis. You can phrase each question in different words and ask if it will heal the damaged area. You can ask if the supplement will reduce the pain as a separate question. (1) Alfalfa, (2) Boswellia, (3) Chondroiton, (4) MSM sulphur, (5) Glucosamine sulphate, or (6) Cat's Claw.

OSTEOPOROSIS

This is a debilitating problem which affects the elderly. One of the main symptoms is loss of height and another is that bones break easily. Osteoporosis is a brittle bone disease which affects the health of many millions of folks each year, causing many broken bones and visits to the hospital casualty department.

Vitamin D is needed to help the body absorb calcium, so fresh air and sunlight are beneficial. Vitamin D is also found in certain fish including kippers, herring, salmon and mackerel, as well as in cod liver oil. It's also found in tinned sardines and eggs.

Magnesium, Zinc, Beta Carotene and Germanium can often be very beneficial, so dowse each one separately and ask if your symptoms would be helped by a supplement of them.

Advice is available from the Osteoporosis Foundation: www.nof.org and also from The American Society of Bone Mineral Research: www.asbrm.org

PAIN RELIEF

It is so easy to reach for the pain killing tablets when a pain makes its presence felt, but many pain killers can damage your stomach. It's worth exploring the field of natural pain relief, which is usually free from side effects.

The trace mineral Germanium is very effective in removing pain and helpful in improving the oxygen supply to an injury.

Dowse and ask if your pain would be reduced by a course of Germanium?

Another useful pill to have in the medicine cupboard is Myrrh. This is anti-inflammatory, anti-fungal and a natural anti-biotic.

For severe pain and as an alternative to morphine, some folks find the Rain Forest pain relief treatment ABT-594, from the Epibatidine Frog, is the answer.[6] Dowse and ask if this unusual and natural medicine will give you pain relief? If you receive a 'Yes' answer then you can ask the pendulum to channel the correct amount of the vibration of this medication to you.

Amputee pain

Amputee pain can, according to many who have been through this traumatic experience, be relieved by Ziconotide. It's a non-addictive pain relief from the Cone Snail and patients don't develop an intolerance.[5] This amazing pain relief is said to be hundreds of times more potent than morphine, so if you or your family members ever suffer this type of extreme pain, dowse and ask your pendulum if Ziconotide MVIIV will bring relief. Again the pendulum can be used to channel this compound. It works by attaching itself to a part of the spinal cord, known as the Dorsal Horn. Nerve cells that convey pain signals from the body to the brain pass through this area of the spinal cord. For those who want a non-addictive pain killer, the Rain Forest seems to be a good source of natural treatments.

Neck pain

Neck pain and neck stiffness are very common – you only have to look at the number of folks who, when reversing their car into a car parking space, cannot turn their neck and head and have to twist their body round to complete the task. The cause of neck pain can be diagnosed with the pendulum; it is possible to establish if the root cause of the pain or stiffness is one of a range of possible problems. Discomfort in this area can come from several different sources, so dowsing will confirm the problem area.

Often the pain is linked to muscle and nerves, caused by sleeping with the head on the wrong height of pillow. Other neck problems can come from the spinal vertebrae. Problems at the top of the spine are very common. Neck problems can also be linked to a shoulder or head injury, as well as whiplash injury, arthritis or fibromyalgia. Dowse the following questions:

1. Is my neck pain caused by sleeping with my head on the wrong height of pillow?
2. Is the height of my computer wrong? Ask if it is too low, and depending on the answer, if it is too high.
3. Does the neck pain come from a shoulder problem?
4. Is the neck pain is caused by spinal wear and tear?
5. Is Arthritis is present in your neck?
6. Will placing an ice pack on the pain for a few minutes several times each day reduce the inflammation?

Shoulder pain

Shoulder pain is one of the most difficult minor ailments to cure as the area is in constant use. There are four tendons in each shoulder and if one of these tendons is over stretched or a nerve is trapped, the alarm bell goes off in the form of pain. Other causes of shoulder pain can be repetitive strain or arthritis in the joint. Deflected pain can come from the spine or from Bursitis, which is a common problem and is diagnosed when inflammation of the bursar occurs. The bursa is the sack of fluid which sits between bones and tendons. When this cushion is worn, it creates pain that can sometimes be eased by an injection.

If your pain does not decrease after you have applied an ice pack several times, it's time to dowse to find the source of the pain.

Dowse and ask the following questions, mentally stating if it is the right or left shoulder which has the problem:

1. Is the pain in your shoulder caused by a spinal problem?
2. Is the pain in your shoulder caused by Bursitis?

3. Do I have a Frozen Shoulder?
4. Is a tendon in my shoulder damaged? If the answer is Yes, you can ask which of the four tendons is damaged.
5. Have I strained a muscle in my shoulder?
6. Is the swelling in my shoulder due to arthritis?

Once you have established the cause of the pain, you can dowse and ask which of the following would be the most beneficial treatment to heal the injury: (1) Chiropractor, (2) Physiotherapist, (3) Osteopath, (4) Bowen Technique, (5) Massage, or (6) Reflexology.

Knee pain

As with the shoulder pain, you can dowse to ask if it is a tendon injury, muscular, bursar, wear and tear, Bakers Cyst, or Osteoarthritis.

Learning from pain

I damaged a tendon in my shoulder many years ago and constantly aggravated the problem by continuing to play golf when the injured area should have been rested. Over the years, people have told me that long term shoulder pain is usually caused by holding on to a problem and that I must let this problem go! This is fine if you are aware of a problem and if you are the type of person who holds on to your problem, but such a sweeping statement cannot apply to everyone.

I agree that people who are very tense and are experiencing lots of worries may hold their shoulder muscles tight, but a muscle relaxant or a supplement of B Complex can often resolve this problem. Dowse and ask if your shoulder pain is caused by tension? Then ask if a supplement of this vitamin would help to release some of the tension in your body? When you are aware of tension in your shoulders, make a conscious effort to relax them. If you don't know how it should feel then tense your shoulders very tightly and be aware of the feeling. When you let them relax, be aware of this difference in feeling.

We often learn from experiencing pain or illness. If I had done as instructed and let go of all my worries, which would have been difficult as my life was fairly worry free, I wouldn't have experienced the wonders of Healing or gained the experience which has enabled me to write this book! Stop and think about illnesses or injuries you have suffered and you will probably realise that the experience has made you stronger and put you in a situation where you met new friends or gained new knowledge about your body. I urge you to explore alternative therapies and medicines when your body has a troublesome problem – there is a whole new world waiting for you to investigate.

Many people will tell you that they learned from their illness. The same thing applies to men and women who fought in the wars. They didn't want to leave their families and go off to fight but after the war, there are good memories as well as bad ones. My father was in the RAF during the war and didn't see his family for two years, which was a common experience for many families. I can remember asking him about the war and being told that there were many good times. He said he would never have experienced the great feeling of comradeship without it.

Patients who have been cured of Cancer or Irritable Bowel Syndrome have often said that they hadn't realised how good life could feel and that being ill had helped them to appreciate life and get things into perspective.

PANIC ATTACKS

It is difficult to find words to describe the panic you feel when you know a panic attack is about to start. You don't know what to do or how to control it.

The Amino Acid GABA is helpful to some folks, so dowse and check if your body is short of it. Also dowse and ask if your body's Glucose Tolerance level is out of balance? If you receive a 'Yes' answer, use the pendulum to correct the balance.

Ask if a supplement of any of the following vitamins or minerals would reduce these attacks: (1) Inositol, (2) Magnesium or (3) Vitamin B Complex.

Perhaps the attacks are linked to a problem in Thyroid activity, CO_2 toxicity or a food allergy? Dowse and ask your pendulum if any of these are responsible for the attacks.

Should you be unable to find a supplement to reduce the panic attacks, perhaps it is time to explore the possibility that the attacks are instigated by Geopathic Stress, electro-magnetic energy or the presence of a spirit in your home. Your pendulum will confirm if you are sleeping over Geopathic Stress energy and if this is the case, you should cleanse your pendulum and ask it to please remove this negative energy from your home. If the panic attacks are caused by a spirit presence then perhaps there is a local medium who can remove the unwelcome spirit. (*You will find lots of information on this subject in my book 'Spirit Rescue'.*) Electro-magnetic energy can also affect your health, so ask your pendulum if your panic attacks are linked to the presence of this energy? Make sure you do not have a computer or television set close to your bed – preferably not in your bedroom at all – and avoid a radio or other electrical equipment close to your pillow.

Dowse and ask if the Feng Shui of your home is bad. Perhaps electro-magnetic fields are bombarding your home from a mobile phone mast or other source. Or is the negative energy from traffic causing the problem?

If your pendulum confirms the Feng Shui is wrong, you can ask if it is coming from outside. If this is confirmed, you can dowse to find which direction it comes from. Once you know the answer, you can hang a small bagua (eight-sided) mirror on the outside of your home, facing the direction of the problem. This mirror has the ability to disperse the negative energy which is approaching your home.

Panic attacks can disrupt your life and cause your nerves to be on edge constantly, so it is important to explore every possible cause, no matter how ridiculous they may seem.

PARKINSON'S DISEASE

Parkinson's disease is a cruel illness caused by a disorder of the person's brain. Symptoms of this neurological disorder include shaking, similar to tremors, and uncontrolled movement. Co-ordination becomes difficult and in many cases walking becomes a nightmare.

This disease is caused when nerve cells in the area of the brain that controls movement of the body's muscles are damaged. Unfortunately this damage is progressive due to a shortage of the brain chemical Dopamine. When this chemical is in short supply, it causes an imbalance and nerve cells cannot send correct messages.

Dowse and ask if the patient's brain is not receiving sufficient Dopamine to keep it working smoothly. Then rephrase the question and ask if the symptoms are linked to a shortage of Dopamine.

If you receive a 'Yes' sign as confirmation and have a good reliable relationship with your pendulum, it may be possible to use the pendulum to top up the level of L'Dopa (*which comes from the Vicia Fava plant*) in the brain. Dowse and ask if extra L'Dopa would be beneficial to the patient? Ask if it would improve, or reduce the symptoms? If you receive positive confirmation but do not have access to this medication, it is possible with the aid of the pendulum to channel some into your body. This is a very short term alternative to taking the prescription drug L Dopa.

A report in 1992 told us that Levo Dopa, which is found naturally in some leguminosae plants of the Vicia Fava (broad bean), is a very effective treatment for the disease. Research results have shown that this plant replenishes a brain deficient of Dopamine.[4] L'Dopa is an amino acid which is missing in the diet of 98% of the entire world's population.

Dowse and ask if the Levo Dopa in this broad bean will reduce the symptoms of this illness? If you receive a Yes sign, you can then use the pendulum to channel the energy vibration of this plant to the patient.

If the brain is short of Dopamine because of a blockage stopping a supply getting to the brain, dowse and ask if a supplement of Serrapeptase would clear the blockage. This amazing pill is a protein digesting enzyme first isolated from the silk worm. It digests dead tissue and clots in the body, as well as scar tissue on nerve sheaths. (*This pill is available on the internet.*)

Ask your pendulum if the patient's body would benefit from a supplement of the Amino Acid Tyrosine? Many sufferers are short of Tyrosine.

Ginkgo Biloba, Selenium and Cat's Claw have all been found beneficial to many sufferers, so dowse each one separately and ask if they would reduce the symptoms or make the patient more comfortable.

There was a lot of publicity in the media when the late Pope took a supplement of Papaya to reduce his symptoms of this illness. According to newspaper articles, the supplement seemed to reduce his symptoms of tremors, poor mobility and slurred speech.[10] Dowse and ask the pendulum if essence of Papaya would be beneficial in reducing the symptoms? This product is available in health shops.

Dowse and ask the pendulum if the patient's brain would benefit from extra Ascorbic Acid? If you receive a 'Yes' answer you can ask the pendulum to channel the correct amount to the brain. Also ask the pendulum if the patient's Glucose Transporter is damaged. If so, you can ask the pendulum to channel healing to the damaged area.

Some research carried out by Jack Lipton and a team of colleagues at the University of Cincinnati has shown that the drug Ecstasy can be a real friend to Parkinson's sufferers. Their results show that Ecstasy boosts the number of dopamine producing cells in the brain and prevents death cells, which is very good news for sufferers.[7]

Another research study has found that farm workers exposed to pesticides were shown to have a 41% higher risk of developing Parkinson's compared to folks who were not exposed.[8] This raises the question 'Can pesticides in the blood create a higher risk of developing an incurable neurological disease?'

On his website, Dr Joseph Mercola reports that a recent study has shown that folks exposed to pesticides are twice as likely to develop Parkinson's disease as those who have not been exposed to these chemicals. So can chemicals in pesticides and bug sprays damage the brain cells that produce Dopamine? Parkinson's disease occurs when the important neurotransmitter Dopamine (a message carrying chemical) is destroyed in the Substantia Nigra area of the brain.[13] Dowse and ask the following questions:

1. Do any chemicals in pesticide damage brain cells?
2. Does the sufferer have a genetic disposition to Parkinson's?
3. Would the sufferer's symptoms be reduced by taking the drug Ecstasy?
4. Has the sufferer ever been a boxer or suffered regular blows to the head?

Research is reporting that those who have been boxers, or received hard knocks on their head, have a 2.5 fold increased risk of developing this illness. If by any chance you have received blows to the head or have been a keen boxer then dowse and ask if knocks to the head instigated the Parkinson's disease.

Sodium Benzoate occurs naturally in very small amounts but is used in a large amount in many soft drinks to prevent mould. That sounds like a very good idea until you hear research results at a British University suggest that this food preservative has the ability to switch off vital parts of the human DNA.

A professor of molecular biology and biotechnology tested the impact of Sodium Benzoate on living yeast cells and found that this preservative was damaging the DNA cells in the mitochondria. This is a very serious fact, as the mitochondria acts as a power station for cells. Damage can lead to cell malfunction and this could lead to Parkinson's disease.

If Sodium Benzoate in soft drinks can seriously damage cells, does this mean that today's children and teenagers (the main consumers of soft drinks) will develop damage in their DNA, and perhaps suffer Parkinson's at an early age? This is a subject that must be explored. Dowse and ask if Sodium Benzoate can disrupt any of the body's cells if regularly consumed? Professor Peter Piper, a UK expert, stated that the preservatives can totally inactivate and knock out cells.

Next, dowse and ask if this preservative can damage DNA if regularly consumed? Ask your pendulum if Sodium Benzoate can damage cells in the human body? If you receive a 'Yes' answer to any of these questions then you know it is time to ban these drinks in your home.[11]

Many chemicals are in the environment and in our diet, but how many folks are aware of the serious effect certain toxic chemicals can have on our health? The Alliance for a Healthy Tomorrow reports that more than one third of the population of the US is suffering from one of a range of chronic diseases including cancer, asthma, infertility, learning and development disabilities, birth defects, endometriosis, diabetes and Parkinson's disease.[16]

Scientific evidence increasingly indicates that the increase in diseases and disorders is linked to toxic chemicals. Most of us already have over one hundred chemicals in our body and the alarming fact is that many of these chemicals have never been adequately tested for their effect on human health. Even more serious is the fact that they have not been tested for the effect of their interaction with other toxic chemicals *already* in our body. Dowse and ask the following questions:

1. Do the toxic chemicals in our body damage our health?
2. Can the interaction between these chemicals affect our health?
3. Does a strong immune system counteract damage from toxic chemicals in our body?

As well as chemicals creating a health problem, there is also the Heavy Metal brigade who are a constant threat to good health. Mercury is a heavy metal known to accumulate in the brain and damage nerve cells. It's also known to be responsible for the presence of free radicals and oxidative damage. If you would like to find out more about amalgam/mercury fillings and their link with this illness, have a look at Bernie Windham's site on the internet. Type in 'Dental Amalgam Fillings Page' and it will open the earth link at the correct page. You will find it extremely interesting reading.[18]

Parkinson's disease is a frighteningly common illness which seems almost impossible to cure so any treatment that helps, no matter how unusual, must be good news. The number of sufferers is growing steadily and there are over 230 branches of this charity in the UK and many other charities around the world.

PROSTATE PROBLEMS

Prostate problems are very annoying and inconvenient but there are many simple treatments and supplements available to help resolve the problem. One supplement favoured in Europe is Prostarbit, made from Rye Grass. Ask at your local health shop for details of other natural products which reduce prostate symptoms.

Dowse and ask if a supplement of Saw Palmetto would help to reduce symptoms. Many sufferers have found relief from this plant, which seems to have the natural ability to shrink a swollen prostate. Horsetail is a diuretic and can be helpful, while Bearberry Tea or Juice is also favoured. Dowse and ask if any of these would be helpful.

If the prostate problem is caused by a slight blockage then ask your pendulum if a course of the enzyme Serrapeptase would clear the blockage. Cranberry Juice can also be a helpful supplement for sufferers of this problem.

RAYNAUD'S DISEASE

Sufferers of Raynaud's disease experience problems in their fingers and toes. The disease affects the arteries at the extremities of the body and creates circulation problems. Ears, fingers, nose and toes can become very cold and turn white in colour, even in summer.

Many sufferers are short of Magnesium, so ask if your body is short of this important mineral? Also ask if your body is short of Vitamins B6 and B12.

Essential Fatty Acids are helpful and oily fish like mackerel and herring help circulation.[17] Ginger is known to heal circulation problems, so dowse and ask if your body would benefit from including more ginger in your diet. Gingko biloba is also helpful for this complaint, so check with your pendulum if it would be beneficial to your health.

RHEUMATOID ARTHRITIS

This painful and restricting complaint affects the joints, causing them to become stiff and swollen. To make matters worse, the joints soon become deformed and very painful. There are several natural treatments for this health problem which are free from side effects and can often dramatically reduce inflammation in the affected joints.

Dr Rex Newnham PhD, DO, ND, BSc, BANT, in his book *Discovering the Cure for Arthritis,* writes about taking Borox, the most common compound of Boron. His pain and swelling were gone within 2 weeks.[3]

This treatment makes a lot of sense as our soil today is depleted of the trace mineral boron. Fortunately, it is available in tablet form from most health shops. Dowse and ask if a supplement of boron would reduce your symptoms of this illness. Also ask if your body is short of calcium as the level of boron affects the working of calcium in the body.

Tests carried out on Green Lipped Mussels in New Zealand showed that they were beneficial in reducing symptoms. Organic Silica is also an excellent treatment for some sufferers, and Devil's Claw tested in China showed 90% of patients greatly reduced joint inflammation.

Check your body to see if the Yin and Yang are balanced. It's common for sufferers to have an imbalance and the pendulum can balance this energy. Also, ask the pendulum if your body would benefit from a supplement of any of the following minerals: Zinc, Magnesium, Calcium, Boron, Manganese, Selenium? Once you have found out which minerals are short, it is time to ask which of the following plants would reduce the symptoms: (1) Dandelion, (2) Agrimony, (3) Cat's Claw, (4) Feverfew, (5) Alfalfa, (6) Glucosamine, (7) Boswellia, or (8) Devil's Claw Root Tea.

Next, ask if the body is short of the Amino Acid Histadine? Boswellia (Frankincense) is a medication with a very long history – there are references to this plant in the Bible. It has been used in Ayurvedic medicine for a great many centuries, which is hardly surprising as this plant is a very powerful pain killer. Dowse and ask if Frankincense will help relieve your pain. It is available in capsule form.

Many sufferers are short of Copper. Copper helps inflammatory conditions so check the level in your body. You can take Copper in pill form but if so, it is important to also take Zinc as they work in conjunction with one another. Alternatively you can wear a Copper bracelet. It's very effective since a high percentage of anything placed on the skin goes into the blood stream.

You may find Celery Juice beneficial as it dissolves acid deposits in the cartilage, which can give relief. Ginger is also useful and Shave Grass can often reduce swelling.

The trace mineral Germanium relieves pain in the hips and improves oxygen supply to the troubled areas. Sulphur has been found to help many sufferers as it cleanses the blood of impurities.

Write down a list of the above remedies and ask your pendulum which ones will be most beneficial in reducing symptoms and in reducing pain. It is also worth asking your pendulum if the Parathyroid gland or Duodenum are out of balance. If you discover an imbalance, ask the pendulum to please balance them.

According to results of clinical trials, Omega 3 fatty acid can improve the symptoms of Rheumatoid Arthritis, while enabling sufferers to reduce their use of non-steroid anti-inflammatory drugs. Dowse and ask your pendulum if a supplement of Omega 3 would reduce the symptoms of this illness?

Rheumatoid Arthritis can be caused by an imbalance in the body's Acid/Alkaline pH level. When too high a level of acid is present, an acid accumulation is created. This causes dryness and irritation in the joints which in turn causes pain and stiffness. If you suffer from any arthritic joints, it is well worth checking your body's acid/alkaline level. Dowse and ask the following questions:

1. Are my arthritic symptoms linked to excess acid in my body?
2. Is the Acid/Alkaline level in my body out of balance?
3. Will more Alkaline food in my diet reduce the symptoms?

It is difficult to keep the balance correct as most folks enjoy more acid foods in their diet; meat, fish, eggs, cakes and biscuits are all acid forming, while fruit and vegetables are alkaline. The motto is therefore familiar to us all: 'Eat more fruit and vegetables'.

Most sufferers of this illness are either sleeping or working over Geopathic Stress energy, so dowse and ask if this is the case and if your pendulum confirms the presence of this unwelcome energy, ask the pendulum to please clear this energy from the building. The presence of this energy will weaken your immune system and stop your body from responding to beneficial treatment.

SCHIZOPHRENIA

Schizophrenia is a nightmare illness for both the sufferer and their family, so any treatment which can help their disturbing symptoms has got to be a great bonus. Sufferers are often short of some of the following, so dowse and ask if a supplement would help them: (1) Zinc, (2) Molybdenum, (3) Manganese, (4) Calcium, or (5) Folic Acid.

The Copper level in sufferers varies, so dowse and ask if the patient's body has excess Copper. If the answer is 'Yes', ask the pendulum to please balance the level of Copper in their body.

It is important to check the level of Histamine in patient's body as this seems to relate to the symptoms – roughly half of patients are found to be short of it, while the other half has an excess. Those with high levels of Histamine can often suffer depression, feel suicidal, be obsessive and have phobias, whereas those with low Histamine are more inclined to suffer hallucinations and paranoia.

Most sufferers will benefit greatly from a supplement of B Vitamins. Swedish tests showed B12 is beneficial, and it's known that B6 Niacin can help to reverse symptoms. Check with your pendulum if the patient would benefit from extra B Vitamins in their diet?

It is worth asking the pendulum to check if the Thyroid Gland is functioning correctly. If the answer is 'No' then ask the pendulum to balance this gland.

There seems to be evidence that the Schizophrenia apparent in one group of young sufferers is linked to their mother having the Herpes Simplex Type 2 virus during pregnancy. According to research at the John Hopkins Children Centre, results showed that the baby is 6 times more likely to develop schizophrenia after puberty, which is a shocking statistic.[12]

A study on red cell membrane fatty acids in patients suffering from this illness showed a serious depletion of both Omega 3 and Omega 6 oils. When patients were given a supplement of concentrated fish oil for six weeks, their symptoms improved significantly. The clinical improvement was related to the increase in the level of Omega 3 in their body.[15]

If any friends or family members suffer from schizophrenia, dowse and ask if their body is short of essential fatty acids? Then ask if they are short of Omega 3? Now ask if their body is short of Omega 6? If you receive a 'Yes' answer, you can either introduce it into their diet or, if that is not practical, you can ask the pendulum to please top up the essential fatty acids to the correct level. This exercise needs to be done regularly, so check each week to find out if the level is correct.

SOME COMMON SKIN COMPLAINTS

Dermatitis

Your skin is the largest organ in your body and needs your attention – when Dermatitis erupts, it's time for action. Dermatitis is different from many other rashes as it only covers small areas which become itchy, red and swollen.

There is a school of thought which suggests that Atopic Dermatitis is linked to mercury in amalgam tooth fillings. When the fillings have been removed, the sufferer experiences rapid relief. Do you have any mercury amalgam fillings? If so, please ask your pendulum if your skin problem is linked to mercury in the tooth fillings. This is another avenue to explore and if your pendulum confirms it is the cause, it's time to find a dentist who specialises in removing these offending fillings. It is important that you do not have several fillings removed on one visit, to avoid the risk of mercury leaking into your mouth.

Have you tried bathing the affected skin with Colloidal Silver, a gentle cleanser that kills bacteria? Dowse and ask if colloidal silver would help to reduce the rash and then dowse and ask if it would help to heal the rash.

Zinc is very healing, so dowse and ask if a supplement of Zinc would be helpful? If you receive a 'Yes' answer then purchase a bottle of Zinc tablets which also contain copper, as too much zinc can cause a depletion of copper in your body.

Echinacea is very good for rebuilding the immune system, so ask your pendulum if a short course of this plant would be helpful? Some folks firmly believe Sharks cartilage is beneficial, so dowse and ask if a supplement of this cartilage would improve the condition?

Contact Dermatitis, caused by a reaction to chemicals in hair products, is a subject we don't hear much about but it's a very common problem. Perhaps folks don't like to mention that they have an itchy head or dermatitis on their scalp. The Allergy Magazine reports that in the UK alone, there are 75,000 known sufferers and of course many others who don't report their symptoms.

Most hair products other than the 'chemical free' brands contain a range of chemicals and hair colour. Some contain the hair dye PPD, which is blamed for skin irritations.[14] If you suffer from an itch, or sore patches on your scalp, dowse and ask if these symptoms are caused by an allergic reaction to ingredients in your hair products?

A high percentage of every chemical you put on your skin goes into your blood, so perhaps it's time for you to consider using organic chemical free products.

Eczema

Eczema is a skin complaint which can cause distress – as well as being unsightly, the rash-like patches of damaged skin are often very itchy, red, flaky and weeping. Trying not to scratch is very frustrating, particularly when children suffer from this rash. Fortunately it is not contagious, although it often runs in families.

Dowse and ask if infantile Eczema is linked to an allergic reaction? If you receive a 'Yes' answer you can then dowse and ask if the infant is allergic to cows milk, dairy products etc. until you find the culprit.

Some research results suggest that Eczema is much more common in children with margarine in their diet than in those who do not eat margarine; researchers found that those who did not eat margarine were free from these skin problems. It is an interesting thought, so dowse and ask if certain brands of margarine can instigate skin complaints in some children.

Eczema on the hands is often linked to using chemicals in everyday use i.e. forgetting to use rubber gloves when washing dishes, domestic cleaners, or using hair shampoo. You can dowse and ask if this is the cause of the problem and then dowse again to discover which brand is causing the skin complaint. Different manufacturers use different amounts of certain chemicals in their products.

To avoid the skin cracking when it gets very dry, use a good moisturiser which has minimum chemical content. You can dowse to ask which brand is most beneficial.

Dowse and ask if any of the following treatments will reduce symptoms?

Marigold cream is available from health shops; it is gentle and protects from harmful bacteria. **Neem oil** is a natural oil with great healing abilities, and **Omega 3 oil** stops the skin from becoming very dry.

As well as those I have suggested, there are several proprietary brands of cream to treat this disturbing skin complaint.

Psoriasis

Psoriasis is not nice. It causes really itchy or sore patches on the skin which are often thick and very red in colour. It appears most often on the feet, hands, knees, elbows but, if you are really unlucky, it can appear on the scalp. Symptoms appear to come and go and stress in your life seems to aggravate it. Some sufferers have had good results from Light Therapy, which is a painless and relaxing treatment.

Psoriasis is thought to be a problem linked to the immune system and there are several plants available which are known to successfully treat these unsightly itchy patches. Tests carried out in Germany showed that Mahonia Aquifolium cream was successful in reducing the unpleasant symptoms, so dowse and ask if the cream from this plant could reduce your symptoms.

Do you enjoy eating fruit? Black grapes are known to be helpful for this complaint, so dowse and ask if they would alleviate the symptoms? Sulphur cleanses the blood and Echinacea builds the immune system, so these basic aids are useful.

Arbor-Vitae the Tree of Life is found to help some sufferers, while fish oil and Vitamin B12 can often bring relief. Germanium can reduce discomfort and Marigold cream can improve the rash. Dowse and ask if any of these items will help your skin problem and also ask your pendulum if eating garlic can aggravate this skin problem.

Sufferers are often told by doctors that there is no cure for this skin complaint, but is this really true? Is Psoriasis perhaps caused by a blockage or infection in the lymphatics? Ask your pendulum this question and if you receive a 'Yes' answer then ask it to please clear the blockage. Next, ask if there is inflammation in the lymphatic system and if it gives a 'Yes' answer, it is time to ask the pendulum to heal the inflammation.

Perhaps there is not a cure for this skin complaint, but there are certainly several things you can explore to make it more comfortable. Bathing the affected skin in a solution of Bicarbonate of Soda is strongly recommended by some sufferers as it reduces the itch and helps to heal the rash. Other users of this cooking ingredient place the dry powder on the skin, which appears to balance the acid/alkaline level. This powder is antifungal and antiseptic so should help to reduce the symptoms.

Shingles

Shingles (*herpes zoster*) is a really unpleasant and painful illness which often does not respond to treatment. It is particularly common in older people. The US National Institute of Health has introduced a vaccine called Zostavax which is available for the over 60's in the US, to reduce the risk of developing this virus. But do we really want any more vaccinations?[1]

Shingles is slow to respond to medicine because it is a disease caused by the chicken pox virus (Varicella – Zoster virus). This crafty virus, fortunately not infectious, remains in the body after Chicken Pox symptoms have long gone. If you develop blisters and feel tingling or itching, your doctor can confirm whether or not it is Shingles. It can appear on your face, your waistline or your head[1] and it's important to strengthen your immune system in order to help your body fight this powerful virus.

Dowse and ask your pendulum if any of the following plants will reduce symptoms of this difficult to treat problem: (1)

198

Echinacea, (2) St John's Wort Hypericum, (3) Cat's Claw, (4) Lemon Balm, (5) Clover, (6) Buttercup Tincture, (7) Lithium Ointment, (8) Capsaicin Cream, (9) Amino Acid Lysine.

Other skin rashes

Rashes are usually a mystery, as they appear without warning and often there is no clue of the cause. This is where dowsing becomes an invaluable tool – you can quickly establish if the rash is infectious or contagious and the pendulum can also confirm if it is German Measles, Measles, Chicken Pox, a heat rash or an allergic reaction.

Perhaps the rash is caused by a plant such as poison ivy. A few weeks ago, I developed a rash on the palm of my hand after I had walked in the woods. Mystified, I tried to recall where I had been and what the cause could be. I realised that I had stood with my hands on the bark of a tree and that was the culprit.

Perhaps your rash is caused by overheating, or an allergy to a certain plant or food. Dowse the following treatments, asking which will be beneficial: (1) Antihistamine tablets or cream, (2) Bathing with Calamine lotion, (3) Cortisone cream or (4) Colloidal Silver.

Old fashioned cures sometimes work very well, so ask your pendulum if bathing in water containing Epsom salts will reduce the symptoms. Baking Soda also cools a rash and will remove inflammation, so dowse and ask if any of these old wives remedies will help to cure the rash?

SLEEP PROBLEMS

Insomnia is a very common sleep problem and there are so many different causes. Whatever the cause, it can leave your nerves on edge and make you feel that you are walking in a daydream. Sleep problems can totally disrupt your life and you don't receive much sympathy!

Some people need a full 8 hours sleep each night, while others find a few hours is sufficient. As well as the number of hours we sleep, the quality of the sleep is important. Why do so many people suffer from disrupted sleep pattern?

If you suffer from a bad sleep pattern or wake up feeling tired then the first priority is to check for the presence of Geopathic Stress (GS) in your bedroom. When your bed is situated over a GS line, your body will be bombarded with negative energy which rises from water deep under the ground and weakens the immune system. It is important to ask your pendulum if you are sleeping over Geopathic Stress. If the answer is 'Yes', ask your pendulum to please remove this energy. Simply hold the pendulum and ask it to please show you the 'Yes' sign when it has been cleared. The task may take a few minutes but the wait is worthwhile. You will find that when this energy has been cleared, your sleep pattern will improve and you will awaken feeling refreshed.

Although Geopathic Stress is one of the main culprits for disturbed sleep, there are many other causes. Dowse any of the following which may be applicable:

1. Is a computer in the room unplugged from the wall? When the plug is switched on, although the computer is switched off it is still giving off electromagnetic rays which can disturb sleep.
2. A digital telephone point close to your bed will disturb sleep while the base of a cordless phone in an adjoining room can also affect sleep because the emf's travel through the wall. Check that your bed is not against that wall.
3. Does drinking Coffee containing caffeine late at night affect sleep?
4. Does drinking alcohol late at night affect the sleep pattern?
5. Does watching TV late at night keep the mind busy and so disrupt sleep?
6. Bedrooms with large mirrors or mirror wardrobe doors are recognised as having bad Feng Shui. It will disrupt sleep if you can see yourself in the mirror when lying in bed. Hanging a net curtain over the mirror will probably resolve the sleep problem.
7. Is your medication affecting your sleep pattern?

If you have dowsed and eliminated any of the above causes and you still have a problem, it is time to look for a cure.

Dowse and ask if your body is short of Melatonin? Then ask if a supplement of Melatonin would improve your sleep problem? Melatonin is on sale in the US but in the UK it can only be purchased on the internet.

Vervain, Valerian Root and Chamomile are all plants which aid a restful night's sleep and have the ability to relax the nerves. A bonus is that they are not addictive. Dowse each one separately and ask if they would improve your quality of sleep.

Good news for some insomniacs is that the makers of Dr Bach's world famous Rescue Remedy have now produced a new Rescue Sleep Remedy. Light sleepers will benefit from using this non-addictive natural flower essence remedy. It will not cause any side effects while enhancing your quality of sleep.

STRESS

Stress is bad for your health and coping with stress is not as easy as it sounds. The only way to avoid feeling the effects is to get rid of negative thoughts and learn the important lesson of giving yourself some time and space.

I agree it's not easy but it's quite amazing how when you become aware of the effect stress is having on your life, you can control it.

A great way to release anger and frustration is to have a 'Punch the Pillow' session, where you take all of your anger out on a pillow. Ask anyone who uses this method and they will tell you how effective it is at getting frustration out of your system!

Your surroundings can create stress, as shape and design play a large part in our emotions. This is the reason we feel strongly about certain colours or designs, and why we like or dislike certain fabrics.

When you are suffering from stress, anxiety or frustration, it is important to let the energy flow smoothly. It's therefore wise to avoid furniture and lamps with sharp angles and choose softer lines when possible. This rule also applies to soft furnishings as curtains with angular patterns never create peaceful energy.

It is possible to dowse the energy of designs of fabric and ask your pendulum if it will create the desired energy in your home. Ask the pendulum if the fabric will balance the energy? You can also ask if it will disrupt the energy. Shape is associated with the left side of the brain and is linked to reason and logic so if this side is disrupted by busy energy, stress is created.

If you are aware of the cause of the stress, perhaps a particularly unpleasant boss or a very noisy neighbour, then you can take action to avoid the situation when possible. However, if you constantly feel stressed but do not know the cause of the stress, where do you start?

A good starting point is to sit down at the table with an A4 lined pad and start writing down everything you can remember that has happened in your life since you were a child that upset you. When you open this thought channel, it's amazing how many incidents come tumbling in – all sorts of events you had totally forgotten about, which at the time had been hurtful. You'll find yourself saying 'Gosh, I'd forgotten about that upset,' but your subconscious memory had not. Perhaps a school teacher gave you a row when you were not to blame for an incident, a boss unfairly criticised you, a child stole your favourite pen or called you rude names. There are many different situations that can leave a lasting impression on your sense of self and you will find so many events to add to the list. Leave the pad on the table for three days and, every time you think of another incident, add it to the list. At the end of those three days it's time to sit down and have a serious look at the list and to mentally ask your Creator to take all these thoughts away. Say goodbye to them as you burn the paper.

Dowse now and ask if these memories have been released from your subconscious mind? Ask if you will now feel lighter?

Sound is at last being seriously recognised as a Healing tool. This is confirmed by the Welcome Trust – the world's largest medical charity. They have started a project to bring together a number of academics and artists to explore the idea of placing music therapy on a more scientific footing. There is ever increasing evidence that certain music can create physical changes in the body and this has been demonstrated in London at the Chelsea and Westminster Hospital. Their staff have found that patients who listen to live music often recover more quickly and require less drugs than those who do not listen to those sounds.[20] Many of us are aware that listening to the right music can bring great physiological benefits, including the reduction of blood pressure, heart rate and hormone related stress.

Meanwhile, violence in doctors' surgeries is on the increase and is causing chaos – 44% of doctors report having been threatened and 22% have actually been assaulted. A pilot project has been launched to measure the beneficial effect of music in waiting rooms in an effort to reduce violence.[19] Music is widely accepted as a powerful tool to calm the emotions and is expected to dissolve tension. Dowse and ask the following:

1. Can relaxing music be an effective tool to reduce your stress?
2. Does relaxing music help your body to relax?
3. Can relaxing music heal strained nerves?

When you feel stress building up in your body, put on your favourite piece of music. It's time to be nice to yourself!

ULCERS

There are many ancient natural treatments for ulcers whether gastric, peptic or leg ulcers, so it is well worth dowsing the following suggestions. They have all helped to successfully heal ulcers.

Gastric ulcers can often be cured by sipping a cup of unsweetened nettle tea every morning and several times during the day. Another helpful tip is eating liquorice, as it lines the stomach. Cat's Claw is also helpful and curcuma root from Java is beneficial to all types of ulcers. Dowse and ask your pendulum if nettle tea, liquorice, cat's claw or curcuma root will help to heal your ulcer? Many sufferers have found that a supplement of MSM sulphur heals the ulcer so dowse and ask if this supplement would be beneficial?

Peptic ulcers have often responded well to a supplement of MSM sulphur and also to supplements of zinc, folic acid, B12 and Vitamin A. A supplement of the amino acid Glutamine may also be beneficial as it has a reputation of helping to heal ulcers. Dowse each one individually and ask if a supplement would heal the ulcer?

A cabbage leaf is a wonderful natural healer. Simply by placing it on the site of the ulcer for several nights, the leaf acts as a poultice, drawing out inflammation. In the case of a leg ulcer, it should be placed over the ulcer each night. You will probably feel it working on the wound.

Cabbage juice is also recommended to treat ulcers, while Manuka honey is another powerful natural healer. Spreading this honey on an open ulcer has been known to work wonders. These are all natural treatments and are normally without side effects, so dowse and ask which treatment would benefit your ulcer.

ZINC DEFICIENCY

Zinc plays an important part in keeping the body's immune system healthy and a zinc deficiency can cause all sorts of health problems. Folks suffering from a serious deficiency of this important nutrient may develop certain warning signals, such as white spots on their finger nails or a nasty skin rash. Hair loss can often be linked to a shortage of this mineral in the diet, so if you suffer from white spots on your finger nails, an unpleasant skin rash or hair loss, it's time to dowse to check if your body is short of zinc.

This mineral is vital in the smooth running of the body's enzyme function. A zinc deficiency can lead to infertility problems and also in certain cases to Night Blindness. In his book Vita-Nutrient Solution, Dr Robert Atkins suggests that lack of zinc is often linked to a wide range of illnesses including psychiatric illnesses such as schizophrenia, heart disease, osteoporosis and certain other health problems. Other research results confirm Dr Atkins statement that a deficiency of zinc can be linked to neurological and neuro-psychiatric illnesses such as depression, dementia, epilepsy, Huntingdon's disease and multiple sclerosis.[2]

If a member of your family suffers from any of the above debilitating illnesses, dowse and ask if they suffer from a deficiency of zinc?

Zinc is long recognised as a reliable treatment for troublesome leg ulcers which can take many months to heal. An old fashioned treatment is to place a paste of zinc oxide on the wound to speed up the healing process. Dowse and ask if this treatment will heal your leg ulcer?

There are many causes of zinc deficiency, including the use of certain medical drugs or excess alcohol! A shortage of zinc can be linked to the level of other minerals in the body with excess copper often being the cause of an imbalance. When taking copper tablets to relieve joint aches I always purchase copper tables which contain a small amount of zinc.

So where is zinc found in the food chain? Zinc is found in many foods, so if you have a balanced diet your body should receive sufficient zinc. However, if your diet is not balanced then by adding any of the following vegetables, nuts or proteins to your diet your zinc level will become balanced: almonds, hazel-nuts, walnuts, carrots, turnips, potatoes, parsley, beans and chicken are among many foods that contain zinc. By dowsing, you can check the level of zinc in your body and establish which foods are most beneficial to retain this important mineral at the correct level for good health.

References

1. National Library of Medicine & National Institute of Health. FDA Consum. Sept. 2006.
2. Dr Robert C. Atkins. M.D. Vita-Nutrient Solution. Simon & Schuster.
3. http://www.regenerativenutrition.com Healing Arthritis & Osteoporosis by Dr Rex Newnham. PhD, DO, ND, BSc, BANT, his book *Discovering The Cure For Arthritis.*

4. International Journal of Alternative & Complimentary Medicine. Sept. 92, by Dan Beth-El. Magic Beans, Natural Sources of L'Dopa in the Treatment of Parkinson's Disease.
5. Medicine Quest page 14 by Mark J. Plotkin PhD. Viking Penguin Group 2000.
6. ibid page 4.
7. Nexus New Times, Vol. 14. No. 1. Jan 2007 Ecstacy for Parkinsons? Source: New Scientist 27th Oct. 2006.
8. MedicineNet.com 'Researchers Say Pesticide Exposure & Head Trauma are Factors in Parkinson's Disease' by Salynn Boyles, WebMD Medical News May 3rd 2007.
9. Journal of Alternative & Complementary Medicine. Sept. 1992. 'Magic Beans' Natural Sources of L'Dopa in the treatment of Parkinson's Disease. By Dan Beth-El.
10. Rod & Pendulum No. 133. July 2003. Brian Hunt. The Daily Telegraph 29th April 2003. Dr James LeFanu's Column.
11. Dr Joseph Mercola 'Drink Soda and Damage Your DNA'. www.mercola.com
12. Nexus New Times, Vol. 11. No. 4, page 37. Frank Strick. Clinical Director, the Research Institute for Infectious Mental Illness. Santa Cruz. 'Micro-Organisms and Mental Illness'.
13. Dr Joseph Mercola, www.mercola.com 'Pesticides May Increase Parkinson's Risk'. Annual Meeting American Academy of Neurology in San Diego, May 2000.
14. Christine Morgan 'Chemical Sensitivity: a Growing Concern,' courtesy of the Alternative Health Magazine. www.alternativehealth.com
15. The Fish Foundation. 'Fatty Acids and Schizophrenia' Lipids 1996. 31; Supp. S163–S165. www.fishfoundation.org.uk
16. Alliance for a Healthy Tomorrow. http://www.clearwateraction.org 'S-1268 & H-2275. The Act for a Healthy Massachusetts; Safer Alternatives to Toxic Chemicals'.
17. Sustainable Life. www.suslife.com 'EPA's Polyunsaturated Essential Fatty Acids – Essential to Health'.
18. Bernie Windham, Editor. 'Dental Amalgam Fillings Page'. http://www.home.earthlink.net
19. Healing Today Oct. 2006. 'GP surgeries experiment with music to alleviate patient aggression'.

MINERALS AND YOUR HEALTH

What is the difference between Macro minerals and Trace minerals? Well, Macro minerals are required in large supplies in the body, whereas with trace minerals (which are a very essential part of good health), only a minute amount is necessary for the smooth running of our system. When a trace mineral is missing in the body, this shortage can cause all sorts of upsets as they are a necessary part of good health.

There are three very separate kingdoms in this world: the animal, vegetable and mineral. Minerals come from rocks and soil and their importance must never be underestimated. This miniscule level can make the difference between good and bad health.

Dowse and ask if your body is short of any important minerals? Then ask if it is short of any trace minerals?

We hear a lot about the importance of having lots of vitamins in our diet, but really vitamins need minerals to create good health. Although our body is capable of manufacturing a few vitamins, it cannot manufacture minerals and these are so essential to maintaining a healthy body.

Minerals and trace minerals are found in many parts of the human body and are vital to both our physical and our mental well being. Most of us would benefit from more of at least one mineral; almost every time I send healing energy to a person, I am told to send at least one mineral. In the case of someone with a heart problem I will be told to send magnesium, with a rheumatic problem I am often asked to send Boron, and with Irritable Bowel problems or Colitis I am told to send Chromium.

207

The interesting thing is that when I've sent the mineral or the patient has taken a supplement of the mineral, their symptoms are rapidly reduced. Again, you must never underestimate the power and importance of minerals in your diet as they play a very important part in keeping your body running smoothly.

While we humans are members of the animal kingdom, we need the vegetable kingdom and the mineral kingdom to maintain good health. All of these kingdoms are meant to interact and we cannot survive without them.

As well as taking minerals in tablet or drink form, it is possible to absorb the valuable minerals through the skin by soaking in water containing these invisible minerals. This is the reason why, for many centuries, people have visited health springs and reported miracle improvements in their health. It's not the water itself that is the cure, it's the minerals contained in the water. Without minerals, the vitamins and proteins in our body are unable to function as minerals are the very basic compounds in the human body.

Here I have listed a few of the minerals which are most helpful in helping the body to fight illness. You can dowse and find which ones are beneficial to you. There are many books available solely on minerals so if you find your body has a serious shortage of any of these important minerals, you may want to explore this fascinating subject further.

BORON

Boron helps the body cope with bone loss and can increase the body's absorption of calcium. It is a real friend to many arthritis sufferers, is very necessary for healthy bones and teeth and plays an important role in the smooth moving of joints. Many arthritis sufferers have found that this trace mineral brings them relief from aching joints.

If you suffer from arthritic type aches and pains, dowse and ask if your body would benefit from a supplement of Boron? Then ask your pendulum if Boron would reduce your pain? Boron is needed to aid the body in it's uptake of calcium to maintain healthy bones and a smooth menopause. This mineral is found in leafy vegetables, fresh fruit, nuts and grains.

CALCIUM

Calcium is needed by the body to build strong bones and joints. It is found in asparagus, almonds, figs, broccoli, cabbage, kelp, prunes, leafy green vegetables, cheese and yoghurt.

CHROMIUM

Chromium is a trace mineral linked to the glucose tolerance factor. When you crave sweet biscuits, listen to your body and dowse to ask if you are deficient in this mineral? Trouble arises when the body is short of this mineral and the body instigates craving to warn us of this deficiency. Chromium Picolinate is available from health shops and is found in meat, shellfish, chicken and Brewers yeast, dairy products, calves liver, cheese and potatoes.

Chromium is a very essential mineral as it enables the body's normal functioning of insulin. Insulin is an important hormone whose job is to assist in transporting blood sugar to cells so that it can be burned to create much needed energy.

As this mineral is involved in the body's glucose tolerance factor (GTF), it should not be taken by Diabetics as they are probably already on medication to control the sugar level in their blood.

Many folks who are overweight suffer from a Chromium shortage, which causes a sugar imbalance and a craving for fattening sweet foods. Perhaps the reason some are overweight is that there is too high a level of carbohydrates in the diet – it is known that high levels of carbohydrates can lead to a shortage of Chromium. In the USA, the FaithMed Institute estimates that 90% of American citizens are short of Chromium in their body.[3] If you are overweight, dowse and ask if a shortage of chromium is linked to your weight problem? This little pill is available in most health shops and is needed by all age groups to balance the blood sugar level.

COBALT

Cobalt is needed in our diet. This mineral is linked to B12 levels in the body and, when the body is very deficient in this mineral, it can play havoc with the levels of B12 vitamin. In serious cases, it can sometimes lead to pernicious anaemia.

Cobalt is an extremely helpful mineral for those folks who suffer from depression. However, before taking this supplement you should dowse and ask if Cobalt would help to lift the depression? Then ask if a supplement of B12 is needed to work in conjunction with this mineral? There can be an interaction between Cobalt and Molybdenum, so it is important to dowse to ask if your body is short of Molybdenum.

COLLOIDAL SILVER

Colloidal Silver is perhaps one of the oldest recognised remedies to fight bacteria – it has been used in history by the Greeks and the Romans. The Victorians and Edwardians used silver food platters and utensils to combat bacteria in food because they realised this was a powerful, non-toxic, natural antibiotic. When hygiene is of utmost importance, Colloidal Silver is the answer. Astronauts learned that fact when NASA used a silver water system in the space shuttle. Following their example, many airlines today use silver water filters.

Before the days of penicillin, many folks used Colloidal Silver as it was free from side effects and was known to kill a wide range of infections. Regenerative Nutrition report in their website that it is known to kill roughly 650 different organisms which is quite amazing when you consider that a modern day, standard antibiotic can only kill up to six different bacteria. Now that so many bacteria are developing immunity to the latest antibiotics, it's time to go back to basics. Colloidal Silver offers the benefits of being natural, non-toxic and completely free from harmful chemicals.

Have a look at Regenerative Nutrition's website for many more details of the magic of colloidal silver. It makes fascinating reading, since this ancient remedy can successfully treat an enormous range of illnesses including those in the following list: Acne, Anthrax, Arthritis, Athlete's Foot, Bladder infection, Blood Poisoning, Cancer, Candida Albicans, Dermatitis, Diabetes, Eczema, Epstein-Barr Virus, Haemorrhoids, Herpes Virus, Impetigo, Lupus, Malaria, Meniere's Disease, Meningitis, Pneumonia, Polio Virus, Prostate disorder, Salmonella, Shingles, Skin Cancer, Staphylo-coccus infection, Syphilis,[1] Whooping Cough and other infections.

Research by Dr Margater Bayer at the Fox Chase Cancer Center in Philadelphia showed Colloidal Silver stopped the spread of Lyme's Disease, which is good news for sufferers of this illness acquired from ticks.[1]

In other words, this amazing natural antibiotic can fight most infections and viruses while being free from side effects. I always keep a bottle of Colloidal Silver in my medicine chest as this inexpensive liquid is a safe treatment to avoid infection in cuts and wounds. It's also useful for eye, ear or throat infections.

Dowse and ask your pendulum the following questions:

1. Is Colloidal Silver a natural antibiotic?
2. Can Colloidal Silver kill certain infections?
3. When you have been bitten by a dog or scratched by a cat will, Colloidal Silver sterilise the skin?
4. Whatever your health problem, dowse and ask if Colloidal Silver will speed up the healing process.

I rate Colloidal Silver very highly. I had proof of its amazing healing powers when a close friend was a passenger in the London Paddington Train Crash. Both of his hands were very severely injured and he was told by the hospital doctors that they would have to remain bandaged for a long time and that he would be permanently scarred.

I sent him Healing and Colloidal Silver to protect against infection and to speed up the healing process. The hospital staff were amazed to find that when the injuries healed, there was no trace of any scarring. I said a silent thank you to this amazing silver for doing such a great job of healing the dreadful injuries.

Doctors in the USA, Switzerland and Canada use forms of silver to treat a wide range of infections. In the USA, it is used in 70% of burns units as it keeps wounds clear of infection. Next time you have an injury or infection think Colloidal Silver and dowse to ask if it will kill the harmful bacteria. This treatment can be purchased in many health shops in liquid form and is a must in every First Aid cabinet.

COPPER

Copper plays an important part in good health as it helps in the formation of bones and red blood cells. It is also needed in the formation of collagen, to help the body to absorb and utilise iron and also very necessary in regenerating blood. Copper bracelets are a favourite with folks suffering from aches and pains. The Copper is absorbed into the blood through the skin and gives relief to pain caused by inflammation.

If you suffer from aches in your body, dowse and ask if you would benefit from extra copper? Also ask if wearing a Copper bracelet would help to relieve the aches?

Should anyone in your family suffer from Schizophrenia, dowse and ask if their body has the correct level of copper? If the level is wrong, it is possible to balance the level with the pendulum. Copper can also be purchased from local health shops and is found in food including beef, shellfish, liver, prunes, leafy green vegetables, avocado pears and nuts. It is also found in water when it has been picked up from the pipes.

The Copper level can be upset by 'The Pill', so if you are using the pill as a contraceptive, dowse and ask if the Copper level in your body is balanced. Copper works against Molybdenum and interacts with Zinc, so it is worth checking that the level of Copper, Molybdenum and Zinc are all correctly balanced.

Excess Copper can sometimes be linked to Zinc deficiency, irritability, Schizophrenia or Dementia while a deficiency of Copper can be linked to nervous system problems, anaemia, or skeletal defects.

Copper is soluble at high temperatures, so hard water can coat copper pipes and protect the occupants from excess copper. However, those living in soft water areas may be more prone to excess copper in their drinking water. If you live in a soft water area please dowse and ask if your body has excess copper and, if so, ask your pendulum to balance the level.

GERMANIUM

Germanium is a trace mineral which plays an important part in good health. It strengthens the immune system and helps to detoxify the body. It is non-toxic and helps the body to fight several different cancers, particularly Lung and Ovarian cancers, as it has the natural oxygen enriching abilities.

IRON

The correct level of iron in your body is important as when this level is low, your energy level also is low. You may also find that your legs ache. Iron is needed by the body for haemoglobin, red blood cells, to strengthen the immune system, for childhood growth and for absorption of Vitamin C. This important mineral can be found in your diet in abundance as it is available in eggs, fish, liver, green vegetables, dried fruit, kelp almonds and avocado pears.

When your body is deficient in iron, your legs may feel heavy, you may develop ridges in your fingernails, brittle hair or constant fatigue and dizziness. If you experience any of these symptoms, it's time to dowse.

Ask your pendulum if your body is short of Iron? If you receive a 'Yes' answer, you should visit your doctor to receive a supplement, or you can ask the pendulum to please top up the level of iron in your body to the correct level. This is only a temporary measure, so it is important to include food containing iron in your diet.

MAGNESIUM

We all require a reasonably large amount of this mineral in our diet to maintain an adequate level of Potassium. This mineral is important in the muscle function of your heart and works to keep it healthy. If you have heart problems, dowse and ask if your body is short of Magnesium?

The right level of Magnesium is important in blood coagulation and a serious deficiency can cause blood clotting. A deficiency of this mineral can also be linked to spasms in the arteries leading to your heart and pains caused by Angina.

Anyone who regularly suffers from convulsions may be short of Magnesium so if a relative suffers from this frightening health problem, dowse and ask if it is linked to a shortage of Magnesium?

Look out if you regularly drink alcohol as you'll lose magnesium in your urine. Also, if you are one of those folks who never seem to have time to cook meals and survive on snacks, toasted sandwiches while not eating green vegetables, then dowse your body's level of Magnesium.

To get a regular supply of this important mineral in your body, get into the habit of eating fruit, green vegetables, lentils, nuts, shellfish, salmon, Brewers yeast, avocado pears, peaches, apples, apricots and dairy food.

Do you regularly suffer from cramp? Unless your cramp is caused by loss of salt due to powerful exercise and excessive sweating, it is probably caused by a shortage of Magnesium in your body. Dowse and ask if a shortage of magnesium is the cause of your cramp? Then ask your pendulum if a supplement of Magnesium would reduce the cramp attacks?

MANGANESE

Manganese is a trace mineral which is necessary for healthy growth and for maintaining a strong nervous system and healthy joints and bones. It's therefore an important supplement for folks who suffer from aches, as it is known to benefits bones and tendons. This mineral is found in coffee, cereal, bran, fruit and nuts, avocado, green leafy vegetables, and egg yolks.

A Manganese deficiency can often be linked to glandular disorders and reproductive problems so if you experience either of these problems, dowse and ask if you are deficient in Manganese.

A deficiency can also be linked to slow hair growth or unexplained weight loss. If either of these symptoms are a problem for you, dowse and ask if there is a deficiency of this mineral?

Your body needs an adequate supply of Manganese as it is necessary for healthy nerves, a healthy immune system and blood sugar regulation. It also works hard to oversee the levels of protein and fat metabolism and bone growth.

Children who regularly suffer from Epilepsy may suffer from a deficiency in the level of Manganese in their body, so if your child suffers from such fits, please dowse and ask if their body is short of this mineral.

MOLYBDENUM

Molybdenum is a trace mineral needed for a healthy metabolism and is found in raw food, organ meat, dark green vegetables and wheat grains. It works to prevent tooth decay and as a real bonus, it's claimed to increase the sexual potency in mature men!

Molybdenum is known to reduce the absorption of Copper, so dowse and check that your body has the correct level of Copper.

MSM – Organic sulphur

MSM is a non-toxic supplement which is very helpful for sufferers of all kinds of illnesses. It's necessary to make collagen and help to repair cartilage and tissue problems. It's also extremely successful in treating airborne allergies such as Hay Fever or allergic Asthma. This medication is also invaluable as a treatment for parasites in the gut, which are often linked to health problems.

I have known many Arthritis sufferers over the years who all swear by their MSM tablets so if you suffer from Arthritis, dowse to ask if your health will benefit from a supplement of MSM Organic Sulphur. It makes a lot of sense, as this supplement cleanses the blood and is involved in the smooth working of the immune system. Whatever your illness, dowse and ask if MSM will reduce your symptoms. MSM Sulphur is found in garlic, eggs, sunflower seeds, lentils and is available in pills from health shops.

When a 15% solution of this organic sulphur is used to bathe the eye, it is known to reverse cataracts and this versatile supplement can also be a great treatment for Emphysema.

In trials, Emphysema patients taking MSM had at least doubled their walking distance within 4 weeks, which is a pretty staggering result for this is a stubborn illness.[2] Dowse and ask the following.

1. Will a course of MSM Organic Sulphur help to improve the symptoms of your Emphysema?
2. Can MSM reduce your Hay Fever symptoms?
3. Can bathing your eye with a solution of MSM reduce the cataract?

SEA SALT

Sea salt is the oldest natural element in the world. It's a natural healer and cleanser and it helps to reduce inflammation in painful tendons. A wonderful cure for sore or tired feet is to soak them in a bowl of sea salt water as the salt draws out any inflammation.

Sea salt is also a wonderful tool to dispel negative energy so, if you know of anyone who is depressed or very negative, then mentally visualise sprinkling sea salt over them. You cannot do any harm and it actually should do some good!

Some healers mentally sprinkle sea salt over countries that are at war to create more positive energy and to weaken the negative energy.

When countries are at war, there is a huge cloud of negative energy overhead that fuels negative thoughts, so mentally sprinkling sea salt and sending the positive thought that it will be effective is sufficient to make it work. You probably don't believe me, so let's dowse!

1. When Sea Salt is mentally sprinkled over a person with the intention of dispersing negative energy, can Sea Salt dispel the negative energy?
2. Can Sea Salt help to create positive energy when mentally sprinkled over countries at war?

SELENIUM

Selenium is essential to human health and is known to cleanse the blood while also being involved in the smooth working of the immune system. This trace mineral and anti-oxidant works to fight off free radicals and protects the body from heavy metals including lead, cadmium, mercury and arsenic. This important anti-oxidant works hard to protect our blood cells, avoiding premature ageing, and helps the body to fight against cancer and heart problems.

Selenium is found in seafood, including herring and tuna, in Brewers yeast and in vegetables. It is often beneficial for children with behaviour problems.

A supplement of Selenium is beneficial to most cancer suffers and it's very easy to include this valuable mineral in your diet, simply by eating Brazil Nuts. Should a member of your family suffer from any form of cancer, dowse and ask if a supplement of Selenium would be beneficial.

ZINC

Zinc is a natural healer. It's necessary for healthy cell growth and speeds the recovery of injuries and wounds. When I was a child, the medication for all wounds was Zinc and Castor Oil ointment.

This amazing cream had the ability to heal wounds quickly and as it was a very thick cream, it also protected from harmful bacteria.

Zinc is involved in the working of the Endocrine glands, so a shortage of Zinc can affect the smooth running of your body. It is found in meat, liver, poultry, shellfish, potatoes and certain vegetables. As Zinc and Copper interact, it is important to dowse and ask if your body is short of Zinc and then ask if it would benefit from a supplement of Zinc? Now ask if the Copper level is correct, as Zinc can interfere with Copper and Iron absorption. Zinc plays an important role in the working of the pancreas by enabling it to produce insulin, so if you suffer from Diabetes dowse and ask if you body is short of Zinc.

SERRAPEPTASE

As there is not a chapter on enzymes, I have included Serrapeptase in the mineral section. It's actually a protein digesting enzyme and was first isolated from the silkworm. This truly amazing pill can digest all dead cell tissue in the body, which opens up a whole new world of treatment for scar tissue sufferers as it can reduce the pain derived from this side effect of operations.

As well as devouring scar tissue, Serrapeptase digests blood clots, cysts and arterial plaque, clears blood vessels, helps varicose veins to shrink or diminish, and is a real friend to those folks suffering from cardiovascular or high blood pressure problems.

It is also an answer to the prayers of folks suffering pain from Arthritis, Lupus and eye problems caused by inflammation. It clears blocked veins, sinuses, fibromyalgia, cystitis and is particularly helpful to MS sufferers as it digests the scar tissue on the nerve sheaths.[1]

Are you wondering why you haven't heard of this amazing enzyme? It is certainly a well kept secret. I only found out by accident when I ordered a bottle after reading about it in a magazine. I have recently started taking a supplement of this amazing pill which has the ability to gobble up scar tissue and already I notice a big improvement in an old back injury, while a damaged tendon is no longer painful (this injury was acquired when my foot went down a rabbit hole!). I have told friends about this amazing pill and they too are impressed with its performance.

DRINKING WATER

We regularly read articles in newspapers and magazines by doctors telling us how important it is for good health to drink lots of water each day, but is our drinking water really fresh?

You can dowse to ask if there are any harmful chemicals in your drinking water and if you receive a 'Yes' answer, you can ask the pendulum to please remove the vibration of the harmful chemicals. You can also dowse and ask the following questions:

1. Are there any harmful bacteria in your drinking water?
2. Does the water contain any unnatural chemicals?
3. Does the water contain fluoride?
4. Does the water contain any heavy metals? If you receive a 'Yes' answer, you can ask separate questions: does it contain Lead? Mercury? Iron?
5. You can also ask your pendulum to please balance the energy of the water and to fill it with Life Force energy.

Water does have a memory and this carries details of all the energy of places it has passed on its journey. Jacque Benveniste did extensive research in France proving that water has a memory and there is an excellent book on the subject called *The Memory of Water* by Michael Schiff. (Thorsons 1995)

We don't know the source of water sold in bottles and most of us don't think about it. Bottled water comes from many sources and is placed in enormous containers.

Things are different in Japan; an enterprising company has purchased icebergs and is bottling and selling this amazing water which has been frozen for 10,000 years. This water will be so incredibly pure – completely free from any pollution or chemicals.

It is possible with the aid of your pendulum to make your drinking water pure simply by asking the pendulum to please cleanse the water of all harmful chemicals, bacteria and negative energy and filling it with Lifeforce. You will be amazed at the difference in taste – I always mentally run light through water and cleanse it before I drink it and am amazed how often folks comment on how wonderful my tap water tastes. Even when dining out I always discreetly cleanse the water. Try it and you'll be pleased you discovered this trick.

References

1. Regenerative Nutrition. Colloidal Silver,.
   http://www.regenerativenutrition.com
2. Regenerative Nutrition, MSM.
   http://www.regenerativenutrition.com Tel. 0845 034 5139.

PLANTS

Today, more and more of us are turning away from conventional medicine and using plants and minerals to treat illnesses. Dowsing is a wonderful tool to help you to diagnose the illness and the most beneficial plant medication.

To say many of us are using alternative medicine is an under-statement. A report by the USA Commission for Alternative & Complimentary Medicine showed that the doors have opened wide on this form of medicine; in America, $17 billion dollars are spent each year on this form of medicine with 158 million Americans using complimentary medicine. The UK is following suit with £115 million pounds being spent on medication, while in Canada 70% of the population have used a form of compli-mentary medicine. Folks in Germany are also enthusiastic about this form of medicine and 90% of the adult population have used a natural remedy. The World Health Organization has reported that the number of doctors now being trained in natural remedy medicine is increasing dramatically.[8]

We often very wrongly think of tribal people living in forests and desolate areas as primitive, but those folks can certainly teach us a lot of lessons when it comes to looking after our health and turning to Mother Nature, who has given us so many plants with the ability to heal our ailments. Alas, our sophisticated lifestyles have led us to ignore this natural approach to medicine and follow the pharmaceutical route. Yes, many medicines do an important job in treating illness, but we must not forget that there are many plants which will treat illnesses and are completely free from side effects. Here I have mentioned a small number of the plants referred to in this book but there are so many other plants which are wonderful medicine for all sorts of ailments.

221

The plant world is a truly amazing place to explore for cures which are free from side effects.

HERBAL MEDICINE

The name Herbal Medicine covers a very wide spectrum of vegetation. It includes very small weeds or flowering plants to large trees. Also in this category are shrubs found in our garden and exotic shrubs from the other side of the world.

Today, cures for cancer and other illnesses are being found in Algae, including the Blue Green variety, and in certain seaweeds and fungus.

Many different parts of these plants are used for medication. Some roots offer great healing powers, while the bark or leaves of some trees are used as remedies for illnesses. Certain seeds and fruit stones are also used as remedies with B17 being a fine example of a cancer treatment found in the stone of the apricot.

Herbal remedies can be taken as a pill or on the skin as an oil, gel or linament and many of these treatments have been used for generations. Ironically, a number of them can be found in our garden. Examples are St John's Wort shrub, with a lovely bright yellow flower, which is a great friend to those suffering from depression. Feverfew plant, with its pretty little white flower, is a recognised cure for migraines while the lovely yellow Dandelion is an excellent diuretic. These are a few of the plants which can improve health problems with absolutely no side effects.

Whatever your health complaint, there is probably an herb which will help to reduce your symptoms. Get dowsing and you'll be glad you explored the world of healing herbs.

If you suffer from Depression, dowse and ask if St John's Wort would help to relieve the problem?

Regular migraine sufferers should dowse to ask if Feverfew would help to control their migraine attacks.

Does your body hold excess water? Dowse and ask if Dandelion would relieve the problem.

AGNUS CASTUS

Agnus Castus is well known as a 'Woman's' plant, as it is rich in the flavonoids and glycocides which help the female body to cope with a hormone imbalance problem. It's a 'must' for those suffering PMT or menopause symptoms – these include the dreaded night sweats, tender breasts and irregular cycles. If you suffer from a hormone imbalance or menopausal symptoms then it's time to dowse and ask the pendulum if a supplement of Agnus Castus will reduce the symptoms?

ALFALFA

Whether sprouting seeds, leaves or tablets, this plant is a popular supplement amongst sufferers of bone or joint problems. This herb is rich in most minerals and is full of good nutrition; it's a source of Chlorophyll, Calcium and Beta Carotene and is known to clear the blood.

The grass is a great supplement for arthritis sufferers as its anti-inflammatory properties enable it to relieve pain. It has been recognised as a treatment for joint pains for many years – I can remember a friend in the Eighties telling me about how she relied on Shakley's Alfalfa to keep her free from arthritic pain, so this is not a new century wonder treatment! If you suffer from Arthritis or joint pains, dowse and ask your pendulum if you would benefit from a supplement of this natural grass? Then ask if a supplement of Alfalfa would reduce the arthritic pain?

Alfalfa is also a great supplement for those suffering from urinary tract infections, bladder, kidney or prostate problems or skeletal and glandular complaints so it's not really surprising that this grass is a great favourite with rabbits. They know instinctively that it contains several vitamins and is good for their health.

If you suffer from a bladder, kidney or prostate problems then dowse and ask your pendulum if a supplement of Alfalfa would improve the symptoms? The nice thing about this grass is that it is free from chemicals and side effects.

APRICOT KERNELS

Apricot kernels have been receiving a lot of media attention recently due to their recognition as a preventative treatment for cancer. They are especially rich in Vitamin 17, which is known as Amygaline and is missing from the Western diet.[3] If you would like to know more about this amazing kernel, have a look at Regenerative Nutrition's website.

BLACK SEED OIL

You may have never heard of Black Seed Oil but it is a supplement well worth remembering. It's truly a miracle cure for many illnesses. Over fourteen hundred years ago, the prophet Mohammad proclaimed that 'Black Seed' heals every disease except death! You can't get a much better recommendation!

So what is so special about Black Seed Oil from other supplements? Well, this extract from the Nigella Satvia plant contains 100 natural chemicals which work together to enhance and strengthen the body's immune system. The healing properties of this plant are many as this amazing oil can relieve pain, dispel worms, prevent cancerous tumours, stimulate digestion, destroy growths of micro-organisms, stimulate bile production and fight viruses, bacteria and allergies.

Black Seed Oil is an antihistamine, anti-bacterial, anti-inflammatory and protects from free radicals. If you would like to find out more about this multi purpose oil, have a look on Regenerative Nutrition's website. www.regenerativenutrition.com

Dowse and ask if a supplement of Black Seed Oil will reduce the symptoms of your illness? Ask your pendulum if a supplement of this oil will be beneficial to your health?

BOSWELLIA

Boswellia (Frankincense) is a plant little known in the West that offers relief to sufferers of painful joints. It is anti inflammatory, anti analgesic and a native of India. It can be purchased as a pill from health shops and also sold as a combination with Chondroiton. I have used this plant with great success for a shoulder injury, so know the benefits of Boswellia.

If you suffer from joint pains, dowse and ask if this plant would relieve your pain?

CABBAGE LEAF

The cabbage leaf is an unlikely treatment for health problems, but this plant has the ability to draw poison from the body and reduce inflammation. It sounds like an unusual treatment but I have used it successfully on a badly sprained wrist and an ankle problem. Each time, it reduced the inflammation. The hard core is removed from the leaf and the leaf is then placed over the wound and held firm by a sock or tape. When I treated my inflamed wrist, I cut the toe off of an old sock and pull it over my wrist to hold the leaf in place. This treatment can be done each night so that it works when you sleep. Cabbage leaf is full of valuable minerals and any type of cabbage can be used.

Anyone suffering from a leg ulcer knows how long these wounds take to heal, so dowse and ask if the cabbage leaf will speed up the healing of the ulcer? You will probably find that by placing a washed cabbage leaf on the wound overnight for several nights, healing time will speed up. This leaf has been used to heal leg ulcers and internal problems for many years.

Dowse and ask if a cabbage leaf placed on the wound will help to heal the leg ulcer? Then dowse and ask if it will be more effective than the present medication?

So what's the secret of this simple treatment given to us by Mother Nature? It was used by the Romans so comes with a good reference. The leaf of the cabbage has the ability to neutralise the cause of the sickness and can penetrate any diseased tissue that may lie unseen underneath the skin. It is really amazing how this leaf works to heal – it's not that the skin on the body absorbs its energy. Instead, it seems to have a natural ability to find poisonous juices and disinfect the wound.

As a child, many of us were often told by our mother to eat our cabbage as it's 'full of goodness,' but few mothers realise the cabbage leaf has other values. As well as containing valuable minerals, it also has healing qualities. These are described by Thomas Haberle, a Benediction Monk, in his book *Helping and Healing*. Another book that teaches us the benefits of cabbage is *The Wonderful Healing Effects of the Cabbage Leaf* by Camille Droz.[6]

CALENDULA

The plant Calendula, commonly called Marigold, is often used to calm stomach ulcers and is an excellent inflammatory treatment for wounds. Calendula is available as a cream from health shops and is a useful addition to the first aid box.

Calendula is also an effective treatment for burns, so dowse and ask your pendulum to confirm the healing powers of Calendula.

CAT'S CLAW

Yet another miracle cure from the Rainforest is Cat's Claw, also known by its Spanish name: 'Una De Gato'. Research has shown that this amazing plant is a real friend to those suffering from a wide range of illnesses including cancer, diabetes, lupus, arthritis and bursitis. The Cat's Claw plant does a great job of stimulating the body's immune system and will help to fight off disease. It is an anti-oxidant that is able to detox the body.

Cat's Claw is a natural anti-inflammatory agent, so it's helpful in healing injuries and is a wonderful supplement for arthritis and bursitis sufferers. This Rain Forest plant is also anti-tumour so is a 'must' for cancer sufferers. It can also reduce the symptoms of Crohn's disease, Irritable Bowel Syndrome and Colitis.

Dowse and ask if Cat's Claw will reduce your symptoms of arthritis. Ask your pendulum if it will help your body to fight the cancer. It is also helpful for lupus sufferers and for genital herpes, so if you suffer from either of these complaints, dowse and ask if this supplement would reduce the symptoms.

This wonderful plant is truly one of Mother Nature's gifts. It's claimed to inhibit thrombosis, prevent strokes and cleanse the bowel, stomach and colon. It also has the ability to lower blood pressure, increase circulation, inhibit blood clots in the vessels of the brain, heart and arteries. Whatever your health problem, dowse and ask your pendulum if your health would benefit from a supplement of Cat's Claw? This Rainforest plant SHOULD NOT BE TAKEN DURING PREGNANCY.

Cat's Claw is available in most Health Food Shops or on the internet.

DANDELION

Dandelion has long been recognised as a diuretic, which is why it's often called 'pea the bed'. This colourful plant contains many valuable minerals and is an excellent tonic for the liver, kidneys and gall bladder problems. It can be purchased as a tea for those who do not want to brew the leaves and root. Dowse and ask if Dandelion tea would benefit your illness.

DEVILS CLAW

Devils Claw is a native of South Africa and a real friend to folks in the West who suffer from all sorts of aches and pains. It is an anti-inflammatory which relieves pain from ligaments, joints and tendons and can be taken as a pill or as a cream which is massaged into the damaged area. I have used Devils Claw both as a cream and as a pill to treat a sprained ankle and found it an excellent remedy.

Dowse and ask if Devil's Claw would help to heal your injury?

ECHINACEA

Echinacea is perhaps the best known and most popular herb on sale today. Over the past twenty years, its popularity has escalated as word has spread of this plant's ability to strengthen the immune system and give it the necessary boost to enable the body to fight infection. I first purchased this herb in 1992 and have been a user since then.

If you suspect that your immune system needs a boost, dowse and ask your pendulum if your immune system would benefit from a course of Echinacea?

FEVERFEW

Many migraine sufferers are very glad they befriended this little plant. Its natural gift to reduce migraine is well known, due to its ability to dilate the blood vessels.

This plant also has an anti-inflammatory action and no side effects. Dowse and ask if a supplement of Feverfew will reduce the number of migraine attacks you suffer?

GARLIC

Many of us use garlic in cooking as it adds a special magic to certain foods but this plant, which has a natural anti-bacterial effect, is also magic to the digestion and cleanses our intestines.

The Allicin in garlic has been shown in research studies reported by the Biochemical Biophysical Act to be an anti-oxidant. Good news for garlic eaters as they receive many health benefits from this plant in their diet; it's also rich in sulphur and is a natural anti-microbial drug with the ability to disable several infectious organisms.

Allicin is also recognised for its ability to prevent heart disease and protect the body's cardio vascular system. An added bonus is the plant's natural ability to make your blood less likely to clot. If you suffer from heart problems, dowse and ask if you would benefit from including more garlic in your diet? Are you one of those folks who cannot stand the smell or taste of garlic? You can purchase capsules from a health store.

Garlic is a real pal to Diabetes sufferers due to its ability to help normalise the patient's body fat, so sufferers, dowse and ask if your heath would benefit from including garlic in your diet? This antioxidant can reduce harmful free radicals, which is great news as these unwelcome toxins can be linked to cancerous tumours, atherosclerosis and ageing.[5] Many centuries ago, Hippocrates recognised that garlic is a natural healer and can benefit many health conditions.

GINGKO BILOBA

Gingko Biloba is a very popular plant in Europe for a range of problems. It is perhaps best known for helping folks improve their memory. As we get older, our short term memory becomes less reliable, so it's ginkgo to the rescue. Gingko is praised by many Dementia and Alzheimer's sufferers as it can reduce symptoms and is known to strengthen the eyes when glaucoma is present.

Dowse and ask if Gingko would improve your memory.

GUARANA

This plant has been used by natives for centuries to successfully treat a wide range of major and minor illnesses including cancer, leukaemia, lupus, fatigue, cramp, depression, bowel problems, severe diarrhoea, digestive problems and heart disease.

Guarana has the ability to thin the blood and is a known anti-clotting agent. Chewing gum containing Guarana is on sale and claims to help adults avoid feeling drowsy. A big problem is that kids have discovered it and love it and some shops are now refusing to sell to children.

There are many internet websites praising the healing powers of Guarana and Michael Van Straten, in his book *Guarana,* reports that it is an effective analgesic, diuretic, decongestant, anti-bacterial and anti-haemorrhagic. This plant is without any doubt 'the patient's friend'.[2]

Dowse and ask if a course of Guarana will reduce your symptoms and then ask if it will be beneficial to your health.

HAWTHORN

Most folks look at the Hawthorn bush in the countryside and don't realise that this flowering berry bush is a powerful remedy for heart problems.

For many centuries, Hawthorn has been recognised as a plant to help regulate heart problems and with the circulation of oxygen and blood to the brain. I recommend this medication to anyone who has a heart problem, unless they suffer from seriously low blood pressure. I have channelled this plant to folks suffering heart problems for many years and found it a reliable medication for cardiovascular problems. Dowse and ask the following.

1. Would a supplement of Hawthorn help with the problem?
2. Can Hawthorn reduce the problems?

The Hawthorn medicine is readily available from herbalists or health shops.

HONEY

Honey is not a plant but, as it comes from plants, I have decided to include it in this chapter. Honey is a natural healer and is used for all sorts of wounds but it looks as though it could soon become a medicine of the past.

The media report that the bee population is in crisis. In the USA, Europe and the UK, bees are deserting their hives and millions of them are not returning home. We can dowse and ask if this is a temporary problem which will soon be resolved. What explanation is offered by the experts for this unexplained behaviour reported by the media far and wide?

These bees seem to literally vanish into the countryside, leaving the queen in the hive. The problem is on a major scale as in the US alone, half of all states are reported to have been affected. The

East Coast has lost 70% of its bee population and the West Coast has fared almost as badly with a loss of 60%.

Many theories have been offered to explain this mass exodus of bees but so far, the scientists have discarded pesticides, mites, global warming and genetically engineered crops. A chink of light is being thrown on the mystery, however; German researchers have for some time shown that the behaviour of bees changes when they are close to overhead power lines.

A study at Germany's Landau University has shown that bees firmly refuse to return to their hive when mobile phones are placed nearby. Are the electromagnetic fields from the phones damaging the frequency of the bees, or perhaps affecting their direction skills and natural homing abilities?[7]

This may be a much more serious problem than it first appears. If the number of bees is greatly reduced then the number of plants and crops pollinated will be greatly reduced also. As crops are a major part of the world's food supply, we could be looking at near famine conditions. It sounds theoretical but this situation could very easily occur in the not too distant future, unless the problem is resolved.

As I work in metaphysics, I have been working with another healer to try to alter the frequency of the bees. The idea is that if they are on a very slightly different vibration, they will not be affected by Electro-Magnetic Frequencies (EMFs). Time will tell if our efforts have been successful – perhaps you would like to dowse and ask if the work we have done on the frequency of the bees has been successful.

Let's get dowsing now on the following questions regarding crops. This problem could have far reaching effects on crops and cattle feed and, at worst, could lead to a massive shortage of food in the not too distant future.

1. Do the EMFs from mobile phones damage the vibration frequency of bees?
2. Do the EMFs from mobile phones damage the bees' homing device?
3. Is pesticide the cause of bees deserting their hives?

4. Are genetically engineered crops the cause of bees deserting their hives?

It is essential that an answer to this problem is found very soon and perhaps we dowsers are better equipped than scientists to quickly find the cause of bees deserting their hives.

As well as food crops being affected, we need the bees to make honey in order to heal wounds. Honey is a natural healer and a natural antibiotic and is used extensively to heal open wounds in many countries. The rapid rise in antibiotic resistant bacteria is encouraging scientists to look elsewhere for alternative remedies to fight these powerful bacteria. It seems to be a case of 'Come back Honey, all is forgiven!' – honey was dropped like a lead balloon when antibiotics came into favour, but now is the time for honey to again be recognised as a powerful tool for fighting bacteria. Honey is a reliable treatment used to treat burns, skin ulcers and open wounds and naturally heals and dries up tissue. As well as being great first aid for wounds, it is an antioxidant which can also act as a sedative to help improve sleep. Even more amazing is that it's reported to help certain cases of bed wetting.

If you suffer from leg ulcers which are slow to heal, then dowse and ask if honey is the answer to this problem. Then ask if a dressing with honey will heal the wound? If you have recently burned your skin, you can dowse and ask if honey would speed up the healing process?

MILK THISTLE

Milk Thistle is truly a gift to sufferers of liver problems. This plant could be your answer to good health as it has been used in many countries as a tonic for the liver for over 2,000 years.

German scientists in 1960 identified a group of active ingredients in this plant called Silymarin, which have the ability to protect the liver by strengthening the outer membranes of liver cells, preventing toxins from entering the cells. It also stimulates protein synthesis in liver cells, which helps to regenerate and repair the liver. In fact, Milk Thistle is known as the best liver protector in the herbal kingdom.[4]

Dowse to ask if Silymarin would help to cure your illness? Then dowse and ask if your body would benefit from taking a course of Milk Thistle?

MISTLETOE

Most of us know Mistletoe as a branch with berries which is hung around the lampshade or in doorways at Christmas, to give us the opportunity to give somebody a Kiss under the Mistletoe. This plant offers many other bonuses.

Mistletoe is a calming herb, renowned for reducing stress and healing the nervous system. It is also a useful herb for treating high blood pressure problems and also hardening of the arteries. Many herbalists use this plant to heal stroke symptoms and it is also known to help reduce cancer. Dowse and ask the following questions:

1. Can a course of Mistletoe reduce my stress problem?
2. Will a supplement of Mistletoe improve my hardening of the arteries?
3. Can a course of Mistletoe reduce my stroke symptoms?
4. Will my health benefit from a course of Mistletoe?

POMEGRANATE

Pomegranate is one of the most beneficial of all edible fruits as it has the ability to protect the body's DNA and protect the liver. It is also known to kill cancer cells and is also an excellent anti-inflammatory treatment. Dowse and ask if regularly eating this fruit will benefit your health and reduce your illness?

RHODODENDRON CAUSASUCUM

This elegant evergreen shrub is found in parts of Russia where it is known as the Georgian Snow Rose and this wonderful plant has the ability to get rid of health damaging free radicals.

It is an excellent treatment for certain eye problems including Glaucoma as it circulates oxygen to the lens and the cornea. It is also known to heal heart disease. I recommend W. Shaffer Fox's book '*100 & Healthy*,' which contains many helpful details of the healing abilities of this shrub.[1]

ST JOHN'S WORT

St John's Wort is a well known treatment for depression due to the relaxing effect it has on the body's entire nervous system. Many sufferers swear by this gentle treatment.

St John's Wort, otherwise known as Hypericum, is an evergreen bush found in many suburban gardens which is used extensively for the treatment of depression. Ask your pendulum if this pretty bush can help to reduce your depression symptoms?

Please bear in mind that if you are on the Birth Control Pill, St John's Wort can reduce its efficacy.

References

1. W. Shaffer Fox, '*100 & Healthy*' Woodland Publishing.
2. *Guarana* Michael Van Straten. C. W. Daniel Company Ltd. 1994.
3. Regenerative Nutrition. http://regenerativenutrition.com Apricot Kernals, a natural way to help prevent cancer.
4. Regenerative Nutrition, Innovative Natural Health Products since 1994. Milk Thistle. http://www.regenerativenutrition.com
5. The Garlic Information Centre, Tel. 01424 892440 'Allicin. Garlic's Magic Bullet' by Peter Josling.
6. *Helping and Healing* by Thomas Haberle. Sheldon Press 1984.
7. Nexus New Times. Vol. 14. No. 4. July 2007. www.nexusmagazine.com The Independent UK 15th April 2007. http://www.independent.co.uk
8. The World Health Organization Fact Sheet No. 134 'What is Traditional Medicine?'
9. Regenerative Nutrition. John Claydon D. Hom. Black Seed Oil. http://www.regenerativenutrition.com

USEFUL INFORMATION

Below I have listed the Code of Ethical Conduct of the British Society of Dowsers so that you can be confident when using the services of one of the Society's members, knowing that they offer an excellent and reliable service and work within the Society's guidelines.

I have also listed the BSD groups in the UK and also international groups so that, wherever you live, you will be able to contact a dowser.

GOOD DOWSING PRACTICE

The Code of Ethical Conduct of the British Society of Dowsers

1. Dowsing Wisely
In your dowsing generally, and when people seek your assistance as a dowser, keep your dowsing focussed on issues of genuine need. Recognise and work within the limits of your competence, and refer to another practitioner or other source if necessary.

2. Dowsing with Respect
Only dowse for information that concerns you personally or that lies within an area of public concern, unless you are asked or given permission by other people to dowse either for them personally or for groups or organisations of which they are members. Do not dowse for information about other people or their concerns without their permission, unless it is clearly in the interest of the highest common good to do so, and do not make unsolicited comments about other people or their concerns based on your dowsing.

Always treat people requesting information about dowsing or who ask you to dowse politely and considerately. When dowsing for others, respect their views, their dignity and their privacy, and protect personal or confidential information of which you may become aware. Explain what you are doing, give your conclusions and advice in a manner that they can understand, and respect their right to consent to or to decline what you offer or advise.

Make sure that your personal beliefs do not prejudice your interactions with other people when you are dowsing, or with the people for whom you dowse – you must not allow your views about anyone's lifestyle, culture, belief, race, colour, gender, sexuality, age, social status or perceived economic worth to prejudice your dowsing.

3. Trustworthy Dowsing

Honest and trustworthy behaviour is expected from every dowser and it is most important that you avoid abusing your position as a dowser.

Be careful not to use your position as a dowser to create or establish improper relationships, either personal or financial. Never misuse privileged information that you may obtain through dowsing. If people seek your assistance as a dowser, be careful to use your dowsing only for their genuine benefit, give guidance and recommendations that you believe to be in their best interests, and share with them all relevant information that you may discover.

4. Providing Information about Dowsing

When providing information about dowsing, it must be factual and verifiable. Avoid sensational or misleading statements, and be mindful of the likely accuracy and completeness of your dowsing as well as of the effects that your information may have on other people as well as on public opinion generally. If dowsing for health or therapies of any kind, you must not offer guarantees of cures, nor exploit people's vulnerability or lack of knowledge, nor put pressure on people to use a service, for example by arousing fear for their future health or well-being.

You must not make claims about the comparative quality of your dowsing nor compare your abilities with those of other dowsers.

5. Respecting Relationships with other Dowsers

Be open and fair with other dowsers, and be willing to consult with them. You must never discriminate unfairly against other dowsers, or allow your views of their lifestyle, culture, belief, race, colour, gender, sexuality, age, or social status to prejudice your relationship with them.

You must not make anyone doubt another dowser's knowledge or skills by making unnecessary or unsustainable comments about them.

6. Financial and Commercial Dealings

You must be honest in any financial and commercial matters relating to your dowsing practice. If you are receiving money for your dowsing you must inform people of all costs before you begin, and you must declare any personal commercial interest in goods or services that you recommend.

7. Legal Issues

You must observe any laws that affect your dowsing and obtain adequate insurance for any aspects of your dowsing practice that requires it.

8. Teaching and Training

The BSD encourages you to continually improve your dowsing knowledge and skills, to help the public to be aware of and understand dowsing, and to contribute to the education and training of other dowsers.

9. The British Society of Dowsers

The British Society of Dowsers exists to provide a forum for dowsers to meet and exchange ideas and experiences, to support and promote good and responsible dowsing, and to provide information about dowsing and dowsers. The BSD Office is always happy to receive calls from dowsers and from members of the public with dowsing related enquiries. We hope that you

Dowsing for Cures

will support the Society, participate in our events, contribute to the Journal, and enjoy a long and fruitful membership with us.

Useful contacts

Anglesey Society of Dowsers
Contact:	Neil Crosby
Address:	20 Trafwll Road, Caergeiliog, Anglesey LL65 3NE
Tel:	01407 740057
Website/Local Groups Page:	http://www.aeriefaerie.co.uk/dewiniodwr/

Bristol Dowsers
Contact:	Jason Viner
Address:	Melville House, 63 Kingston Road, Southville, Bristol BS3 1DS
Tel:	0117 9498933
Website/Local Groups Page:	http://beehive.thisisbristol.com/bristoldowsers

Devon Dowsers (Eggesford)
Contact:	Mr Stephen Elliston
Address:	Ashcroft, Woodtown, Fairy Cross, Bideford EX39 5BZ
Website/Local Groups Page:	http://beehive.thisisnorthdevon.co.uk/default.asp?WCI=SiteHome&ID=2231

Dowsing Research Group
Contact:	Mrs Jo Cartmale
Address:	16 Woodland Walk, Billing Lane, Northampton NN3 5NS
Tel:	01604 646472
Website/Local Groups Page:	http://www.britishdowsers.org/whats on/dowsingjesearch group.shtml

East Midlands Group (Bramcote, Nottingham)
Contact:	Marilyn Wright
Address:	107 Beacon Hill Road, Newark, Notts NG24 2JN
Tel:	01636 672516
Website/Local Groups Page:	http://www.eastmidsdowsers.co.uk/

Greater Manchester Dowsers
Address:	5 Sunnymede Vale, Holcombe Brook, Ramsbottom, Bury, Lancs BL0 9RR
Tel:	01204 883482
Website/Local Groups Page:	http://www.britishdowsers.org/whats_on/g_manchester_dg_events.shtml

Hampshire Dowsers (Lower Froyle)

Contact:	Alan K Barsby
Address:	Larkswood, Holly Close, Eversley, Hampshire RG27 0PH
Tel:	0118 973 2478
Website/Local Groups Page:	http://www.britishdowsers.org/whats_on/ hampshire_dg_events.shtml

Kent Dowsers Group

Contact:	Rob MacManaway
Address:	32 Court Lane, Hadlow, Kent TN11 0DU
Tel:	01732 851520
Website/Local Groups Page:	http://www.britishdowsers.org/whats_on/ kent_dg_events.shtml

London & Thameside Dowsers (Mile End)

Contact:	Vicky Sweetlove
Address:	8 Rayleigh Road, Hutton, Brentwood, Essex CM13 1AE
Tel:	01277 203180
Website/Local Groups Page:	http://www.londondowsers.org/

Malvern Dowsers (Great Malvern, N Herefords & Worcester)

Contact:	Ced Jackson
Address:	3 Ebrington Road, West Malvern, Worcs WR14 4NL
Tel:	01684 560265
Website/Local Groups Page:	http://www.fengshuifutures.com/mdindex.htm

New Forest Dowsers Society (Ringwood, Hants)

Contact:	Mr David Webb
Address:	10 Castle Dene Lodge, 31 Throop Road, Bournemouth, Dorset BH8 0BY
Website/Local Groups Page:	http://www.britishdowsers.org/whats_on/ newforest_dg_events.shtml

Northamptonshire Dowsers (Moulton)

Contact:	Maureen Clarke
Address:	The Cottage, Forest Road, Long Street, Hanslope, Milton Keynes, MK19 7DE
Tel:	01908 510379
Website/Local Groups Page:	http://www.northamptondowsers.co.uk/

Senlac Dowsers (St Leonards on Sea)

Contact:	Jim Harrison
Address:	The Pinehurst Centre, 3 Avondale Road, St Leonards-on-sea TN38 0SA
Tel:	07927 723730
Website/Local Groups Page:	http://www.britishdowsers.org/whats_on/ senlac_dg_events.shtml

Slimbridge Dowsing Group
Contact:	Peter Golding
Address:	Little Kingston, Moorend Lane, Slimbridge, Gloucester GL2 7DG
Website/Local Groups Page:	http://www.petergolding.net/HTML/slimbridge.html

Scottish Dowsing Association
Contact:	Mr G Harper
Address:	14 Scott Drive, Largs, Ayrshire KA30 9PA
Tel:	01475 674364

South Herefordshire Dowsers
Contact:	David Exell
Address:	1 Saxon Way, Ledbury, Herefordshire HR8 2QY
Tel:	01600 716115
Website/Local Groups Page:	http://www.dowsers.org.uk/

South Coast Dowsers
Contact:	Paul Craddock
Address:	6 Library Road Parkstone, Poole, Dorset BH12 2BE
Tel:	0870 4280934
Website/Local Groups Page:	http://www.healthyandwise.co.uk/south_coast_dowsers.htm

South Wales Dowsers
Contact:	Irenka Herbert
Address:	The Newport Clinic of Holistic Health, 4 Llanthewy Road, Newport NP20 3RJ
Tel:	01633 843333
Website/Local Groups Page:	http://www.britishdowsers.org/whats_on/south_wales_dowsers_events.shtml

Surrey Dowsers
Contact:	Joan Meech
Address:	17 Greenfield Avenue, Surbiton, Surrey KT5 9HP
Tel:	020 8399 9367
Website/Local Groups Page:	http://www.surreydowsers.org.uk/

Sussex Dowsers (Chichester)
Contact:	Mrs Jo Caulfield
Address:	75 North Road, Portslade, Brighton, E Sussex BN41 2HD
Tel:	01273 422391
Website/Local Groups Page:	http://www.britishdowsers.org/whats_on/sussex_dowsers events.shtml
Email:	smcken@btopenworld.com

Useful Information

Tamar Dowsers
Contact: Jacki Ellis-Martin
Address: Glenkeller, 10 Dutson Road, Launceston,
Cornwall PL15 8DY
Tel: 01566 774902
Website/Local Groups Page: http://www.tamar-dowsers.co.uk/

Thames Valley Dowsers
Contact: Sue Scott Powell
Address: Jubilee Cottage, Nursery Lane, Penn, Bucks HP10 8LT
Tel: 01494 813214
Website/Local Groups Page: http://www.britishdowsers.org/whats_on/
thames_dg events.shtml

Wessex Dowsers (Wareham)
Contact: Mrs Chris Burgess
Address: 6 Bestwall Road, Wareham, Dorset BH20 4HZ
Tel: 01929 551539
Website/Local Groups Page: http://www.wessexdowsers.co.uk

West of Scotland Dowsers (Glasgow)
Contact: Catherine Kirk
Address: 53 Hamilton Drive, Glasgow G12 8DP
Tel: 0141-339 0678
Website/Local Groups Page: http://www.britishdowsers.org/whats_on/
west_scotland_dg_events.shtml

West Midland Dowsers
Contact: Mr M Guest
Address: 25 Calthorpe Close, Walsall, West Midlands WS5 3LT
Tel: 0121 357 1117
Website/Local Groups Page: http://www.britishdowsers.org/whats_on/
west_midlands_dg_events.shtml

West Wales Dowsers Society
Contact: Ros Briagha
Address: Elfane, Mynyddcerrig, Nr Llanelli,
Carmarthanshire SA15 5BD
Tel: 01269 870175
Website/Local Groups Page: http://www.westwalesdowsers.co.uk/

Wyvern Dowsing Society
Contact: Mrs Sara Daw
Address: 8 Orchard Road, Marlborough, Wilts SN8 4AU
Tel: 01672 515673
Website/Local Groups Page: http://www.wyverndowsing.freeserve.co.uk/

The American Society of Dowsers
Address: Danville, Vermont 05828, USA
Tel: 001 802 684 3417
Fax: 001 802 684 2565
Website:
Email:

Association Argentina de Radiestesia
Address: Juan Carlos Russo
                           A Jauretche, 75 (1405) Buenos Aires, Argentina
Tel: 0054 11 4 982 7159
Website: www.radiestesiaargentina.netfirms.com
Email: radiestesiadeargentina@fibertel.com.ar

Dowsers Society of New South Wales Inc
Address: 7 Maycock Street, Denistone East, NSW 2113, Australia
Tel:
Website:
Email:

Dowsers' Club of S Australia Inc
Address: PO Box 2427, Kent Town 5071, South Australia
Website:
Email:

Dowsing Society of Victoria Inc
Address: PO Box 4278, Ringwood, Victoria 3134, Australia
Tel: www.dsv.org.au
Website: http://www.eastmidsdowsers.co.uk/
Email: lyn.wood@optusnet.com.au

North Tasmania Dowsing Association
Address: 2515 West Tamar Highway, Exeter, Tasmania 7275, Australia
Tel:
Website:
Email:

South Tasmania Dowsing Association
Address: PO Box 530, Moonah, Tasmania 7009, Australia
Tel:
Website:
Email:

Osterreichischer Verband für Radiasthesie und Geobiologie
Address: Florianigasse 43/1/12, A-1080, Vienna, Austria
Tel:
Website:
Email:

Useful Information

Belgian-Dutch LA Dowsers Association

Address:
Mrs N Leunens
Ninoofsesteenweg 91 1500 Halle, Belgium

Tel:
Website:
Email:

Canadian Society of Dowsers

Address:
7-800 Queenston Road, Suite 152, Stoney Creek,
Ontario L8G 1A7, Canada

Tel:
1-888-588-8958

Website:
www.canadiandowsers.org

Email:
susanjcollins@rogers.com

Toronto Dowsers

Contact:
Marilyn Gang

Address:
816-225 Davisville Avenue, Toronto,
Ontario M4S 1G9, Canada

Tel:
(416) 322-0363

Website:
www.TorontoDowsers.com

Email:
mgang@dowsers.info

The Canadian Society of Questers

Address:
PO Box 4873, Vancouver B.C., Canada V6B 4A6

Tel:
01424 423687

Website:
www.questers.ca

Centro Latino Americano de Parapsicologia

Contact:
Eng Carlos Freire

Address:
Rua Joao Moura, 591 Jardim America,
CEP 05412-001, San Paulo, Brazil

Tel:
0**11 3891 0465

Website:
www.radiestesiaonline.com.br
www.abrad.com.br

Email:
pauloa@abrad.com.br

Dowsing Society of Chile

Contact:
Juan Guillermo Prado

Address:
Londres 65, Santiago del Chile,
Republica de Chile, South America

Tel:
2 201 33 82

Website:
www.sociedadradiestesia

Email:
jprado@bcn.cl

Scientific International Union of Dowsing

Address:
Via Blanca y Carretera Central, San Miguel del Padrón,
C. Habana, Cuba CP 11000

Tel:
537 557232

Email:
igpcnig@ceniai.inf.cl

Miljf- & Jordstraleforeningen Danmark
Address: Henning Juhl
            Grænsevej 49, DK 2650 Hvidovre Copenhagen,
            Denmark

Les Amis de la Radiesthésie
Contact: François Ferval-Chanut
Address: 9 rue Larrey, 75005 Paris, France
Tel: 00 33 1 45 35 54 77

Syndicat National des Radiesthésistes
Address: 21 boulevard de la Libération, 94300 Vincennes,
            France
Tel: 00 33 1 41 93 06 31

Herold-Verlag Dr Wetzel
Address: Kirchbachweg 16, 81479 München, Germany

Indian Society of Dowsers
Contact: Arun Patel (President)
Address: 81/961 Shreenath apartment, Nr Vayash Wadi,
            Nava Vadaj Ahemadabad 380 013, Gujarat, India
Email: arunpatel_ohm@yahoo.com

Irish Society of Diviners
Contact: Joe Mullally
Address: ANAM, Manor Kilbride, Blessington, Co Wicklow,
            Irish Republic
Tel: 01 285 9954
Email: earthwise@tinet.ie

Japanese Society Of Dowsers
Contact: Yuji Tsutsumi
Address: Room 202 Nagao-so, 3-24-19 Nakamachi Koganei-city,
            Tokyo 184, Japan

The Korean Society of Dowsers
Contact: Mr Dea Hoon Kang
Address: 220-507 Ju Gong A P T, TaeHyung-Dong,
            Jung-Gu Daejeon City, Korea
Tel: 00 82 042 634 8227/8
Email: HD111@chollian.net

Baltic Dowsers Association
Address: Latvian Academy of Sciences, Institute of Physics,
            Salaspils-1, LV-2 169, Latvia

Useful Information

Nederlands Genootschap voor Radiësthésue en Radionica
Address: H W J den Hartog
Postbus 44, 1440 AA Purmerend, The Netherlands

New Zealand Society of Dowsing & Radionics Inc
Address: PO Box 41-095, St Lukes, Auckland 3,
New Zealand

Norwegian Society of Dowsers
Address: (Norsk Kuistgjenger-forening), v/Geir A B Wollmann,
Zinoberveien, N-0758 Oslo, Norway

Associaçao Cultural Radiestesia Lusitaniae
Contact: Alexander Cotta
Address: PO Box 41-095, St Lukes, Auckland 3, New Zealand
Tel: (351) 2 600 2341
Website: www.acrl.web.pt
Email: info@acrl.web.pt

Central Ustugowo Wytworcza 'Rodzkarz'
Address: ul Zbaszynska 28, 60 359 Poznan, Poland

Stowarzyszenie Radiestetow w Warszawie
Address: Ul Noakowskiego 10 m 54, 00-666 Warszawa, Poland

Russian Association of Dowsers
Contact: Akim Bogatyrev
Address: leningradskoe shosse d9 korp3 rv516,
Moscow 125171, Russia
Email: akim-tonic@mtu-net.ru

Sociedad Espanola de Parapsicologia
Address: Valentin Robledo 21, Pozuelo de Arcon, Madrid, Spain

Svenska Slagruteforbundet
Address: Stockholmsv. 158, 187 32 Taby, Sweden
Tel: 8-758 55 90
Website: www.slagruta.org

Jordstralningscentrum
Address: Stockholmsv. 158, 187 32 Taby, Sweden
Tel: 8-510 110 25
Website: www.jordstralningscentrum.nu

Swiss Association of Radiästhesie
Contact: Mr G Heer
Address: Hermenweg 3, CH-5702 Niederlenz,
Switzerland

Centre of Eniology

Address:	Ternopolska ST, 3/33, Lviv 79034, Ukraine
Tel:	00 380 0322 70 59 92
Email:	oturkot@ukr.net

Instituto de Filosofia y Parapsicologia Jofralena

Address: Apartado 40.472 Zona Postal 1040-A,
Nueva Granada, Caracas, Venezuela

Jakarta Society of Dowsers

Address: Jalan Gading Indah Utara II, NH3 N0.1
Kelapa Gading Permai, Utara 14250, Jakarta